sister vegetarian's

31 DAYS OF DRAMA-FREE LIVING

sister vegetarian's

31 DAYS OF DRAMA-FREE LIVING

Exercises and Recipes for a
Healthy Mind, Body, and Spirit

DONNA M. BEAUDOIN

LANTERN BOOKS • NEW YORK • A DIVISION OF BOOKLIGHT INC.

2012
Lantern Books
128 Second Place
Brooklyn, NY 11231
www.lanternbooks.com

Printed in the United States of America

Library of Congress Cataloging-in-Publication Data

Beaudoin, Donna M.
Sister Vegetarian's 31 days of drama-free living : exercises and recipes for a healthy mind, body, and spirit /
Donna M. Beaudoin.
p. cm.
ISBN 978-1-59056-318-2 (alk. paper) — ISBN 978-1-59056-319-9 (ebook)
1. Vegetarianism. 2. Personal health. 3. Exercise. 4. Nutrition. I. Title. II. Title: 31 days of drama-free living.
III. Title: Sister Vegetarian's thirty-one days of drama-free living.
TX391.B43 2012
641.5'636—dc23

2011032109

Print ISBN: 9781590563182
Ebook ISBN: 9781590563199

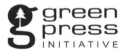

Lantern Books has elected to print this title on Rolland Enviro, a 100% post-consumer
recycled paper, processed chlorine-free. As a result, we have saved the following resources:

10 trees, 1,223 lbs of solid waste, 7,671 gallons of water
15 million BTUs, and 3,178 lbs of greenhouse gases

As part of Lantern Books' commitment to the environment we have joined the Green Press Initiative,
a non-profit organization supporting publishers in using fiber that is not sourced from ancient or
endangered forests. We hope that you, the reader, will support Lantern and GPI in our endeavor to
preserve the ancient forests and the natural systems on which all life depends. One way is to buy books
that cost a little more but make a positive commitment to the environment no only in their words, but in
the paper that they are published on. For more information, visit www.greenpressinitiative.org.

contents

Acknowledgments 11

How to Use This Book as a Daily Guide 13

*"Encourage Yourself"—A Poem of Inspiration
to Get You Started on Your Way by Tashi S. Winston* 21

DAY 1: VICTORY! 23

Recipe: Victory! I Am Alive and
Well Curried Raw Beet Greens Salad 26

DAY 2: GOALS CAN HELP YOU MAINTAIN A VEGETARIAN LIFESTYLE 32

Recipe: Just Like Grandma Vegan
Cinnamon-Raisin Wheat Bread 35

DAY 3: TIRED OF BEING SICK AND TIRED (MY STORY) 39

Recipe: Sick No More Curried Split-pea Soup
with Sweet Potatoes and Mustard Greens 43

DAY 4: BECOME AN ACTIVIST FOR CHANGE BY TALKING TO YOUR LOCAL GROCERY STORE 47

Recipe: Nathaniel Gaskins' Sixteen Bean Soup 50

DAY 5: TAKE A STEP OF FAITH 53

Recipe: Vegan-style Huevos Rancheros (Scrambled Tofu Topped with Cuban Aioli Spicy Avocado Sauce) 55

DAY 6: WE COME IN ALL SIZES 59

Recipe: Breakfast of Champions 61

DAY 7: CONGRATULATIONS! ONE FULL WEEK COMPLETED! 64

Recipe: Celebration Black-eyed Peas Stew 66

DAY 8: YES, YOU WILL CRAVE MEAT 69

Recipe: Uncle Joe's Cuban Sandwich 73

DAY 9: HEY . . . GOOD LOOKIN' 76

Recipe: Spicy Mexican Cornbread 79

DAY 10: YES, YOU CAN STILL HAVE A FLY AND PHAT ASS 81

Recipe: Fly and Phat Collard Greens Hummus Wrap 84

DAY 11: COURAGE 87

Recipe: Courageous Spicy-Smoky Beet Hummus 90

DAY 12: DON'T MESS WITH MY MIND   92

Recipe: Don't Mess with My Pesto!   95

DAY 13: UNIQUE AND PROUD   98

Recipes: Great-grandma's Proud Virginia
Diner Chunky Vegetarian Chili   101

DAY 14: KEEP IT SIMPLE   103

Recipe: Simple After-work Sautéed Beets
and Garlic Served over Pasta and Greens   105

**DAY 15: YOUR FAMILY MAY NOT ALWAYS
BE SUPPORTIVE, BUT THAT'S OKAY**   108

Recipe: *La Familia* Cuban Black Bean Soup   111

DAY 16: SOAR UPHILL!   114

Recipe: Energizing Tortilla Pinto Bean Wrap   116

DAY 17: REWARDS OF CLEAR SKIN   118

Recipe: Water As I Rise   121

DAY 18: VEGETARIANISM OFFERS FUEL FOR THE BODY   123

Recipe: Fuel Me Kushari   126

DAY 19: STEP OUTSIDE THE BOX   129

Recipe: Sweet Potato French Fries   132

DAY 20: COOKING LIKE THE PROS   134

Recipe: Cooking Like the Pros Fusion Pad Thai   137

**DAY 21: THREE WEEKS OF DRAMA-FREE
VEGETARIAN LIVING: PRAISE YOURSELF!**   140

Recipe: Celebration Grilled Acorn Squash Salad   143

DAY 22: BE A CHILD AGAIN   146

Recipe: The Child in Me Veggie Burger   149

DAY 23: I AM NOT AFRAID   152

Recipe: I'm Not Afraid Calzone   155

DAY 24: SECOND CHANCE AT LIFE   158

Recipe: Second Chance Cold Vegetable Wrap   159

DAY 25: BREATHE DEEP AND RELAX   161

Recipe: Breathe Deep Herbal Ice Tea   164

DAY 26: IT ALL HAS TO DO WITH THE INDIVIDUAL JOURNEY   166

Recipe: Individual Falafel Journey   169

DAY 27: CALLING UPON OUR LIFE FORCE   172

Recipe: I Am Chole Palak   175

DAY 28: FOUR WEEKS OF VEGETARIAN LIVING 178

Recipe: You Can Do It Chapati Bread 180

DAY 29: ALWAYS SMILE 183

Recipe: Make Me Smile Spicy-Chunky
Spanish Gazpacho Soup 185

**DAY 30: CONGRATULATIONS! A SUMMARY OF DRAMA-FREE
MIND, BODY, AND SPIRIT VEGETARIAN LIVING** 187

Recipe: On Another Journey Sautéed Heirloom Vegetables 189

DAY 31 LIVE LONG AND PROSPER 191

Sister Vegetarian's Energy Bars 192
Recipe: Red Quinoa, Lentils, and Farro Cakes,
by Chef Ricky Moore 197

*Rights of Passage Reborn—
A Poem of Motivation to Keep Going Farther by Tashi S. Winston* 201

Appendix I: What's in Sister Vegetarian's Pantry? 203

Appendix II: Additional Resources: Documentaries and Books 207

Appendix III: Sister Vegetarian's Drama-free Goals Chart 211

Appendix IV: Sister's Weekly Meal Planner 213

acknowledgments

I would like to express my gratitude to and appreciation for the many individuals who made this book grow from a thought to reality. In the words of Napoleon Hill, "What the mind of man can conceive and believe, it can achieve."

Thank you, God, for providing me with the dream, idea, and talent to inspire and motivate others to lead a vegetarian or vegan lifestyle, and to Mother Earth for providing the nourishment, fuel, and nutrients we need to live strong, healthy, active, and vibrant lives.

Thanks also to my friends of thirty-plus years, Kathy and Karen Breeden (aka the Breeden Twins), who've known me since junior high, when I'd bring healthy vegetarian and raw vegan lunches to school, and who told me I should write a book of my vegetarian experiences. The Twins provided the daily kick in the butt I needed never to give up on this dream. They saw what I could do and become when I didn't see it for myself.

Thanks to my maternal great-grandmother, Otis Mae Robinson, who lived to be a hundred years old by incorporating vegetarian meals into her lifestyle. She continued to be strong and active in her community until she parted the Earth. I miss her.

Thanks to my mother, Edith Fomby Gibbons, who introduced me to beets, eggplant, various beans, greens, and many other vegetables when I was a toddler. She proved that children will eat all types of vegetables if you show them the beauty of Mother Earth's natural products. Mom: Do you remember the poem I wrote at age twelve, where the first lines stated, "Who am I? What will I become? / A writer writing with the stroke of my black pen?" I know you still have that poem as a keepsake.

Thanks to my father, Donald Gibbons, for the books he brought home and which fostered my love of reading and writing, which began before I was five years old. He was the catalyst that kept me writing through the years.

Thanks to my husband, Patrick. He's my soul mate and best friend, and was patient and understanding as I took time away to write this book. I did it!

Thanks to those who served as mentors, without even knowing it: Trayce McQuirter of *By Any Greens Necessary*, A. Breeze Harper of *Sistah Vegan*, and Martha Theus of 21st Century Vegetarian. Ladies, you are my inspiration. I'm honored that the three of you took the time to converse with me when Sister Vegetarian's blog was in its infancy.

Thank you, Sister Vegetarian's reader and poster, Aby "Battzi" Rhys. Thank you for bringing others to the blog and sharing weekly updates on your vegan journey. Readers like you were my inspiration to encourage others to stay on this healthy path.

Finally, thank you Sister Vegetarian's readers and contributors! This book is for—and about—you. May you be inspired, motivated, empowered, encouraged, and *victorious* in this journey!

how to use this book as a daily guide

"I am sick and tired of being sick and tired."
—FANNIE LOU HAMER, CIVIL RIGHTS ACTIVIST

I felt like Fannie Lou Hamer. I was sick and tired of all the stomach and colon ailments I experienced when I ate meat. I was sick and tired of being hospitalized for belly pain and the accompanying vomiting that the physicians couldn't figure out the cause for. I was sick and tired of catching colds and viral infections every couple of months. I was sick and tired of seeing relatives, friends, and acquaintances passing before their time, or even hearing the television news reporting on someone dying young.

I looked at the woman in the mirror, and saw someone who was sick and tired of being sick and tired of illnesses arising from the foods I ate. I knew that, unless I made a change in how I lived, I was a potential candidate for the diabetes, heart disease, and colon and stomach cancers that had plagued both sides of my family. I knew that becoming a vegetarian[1]

---

1   For the sake of brevity, rather than using "vegetarian and vegan" constantly in the book, I use the word "vegetarian" for each day's inspirations. Nonetheless, this book applies both to vegetarians (who consume dairy, eggs, and cheese) and vegans (who don't eat any animal products).

(and, even more, a vegan) could have made all the difference to them, and I knew the same for myself. I wanted everyone, whether I was related to them or not, to be the walking living and not the barely walking dead. I was ready to be alive and well! I needed to become a vegetarian.

Nonetheless, I found becoming—and, more significantly, remaining— meat-free very hard. I wasn't alone. Coworkers and newbie vegetarians would exclaim how difficult it was to maintain a vegetarian lifestyle, and how they'd give up almost as soon as they started. Many would transition for months, and then just never begin; others would go cold turkey, as I did, and then start eating meat within a month, or six months, or a year. I even read on a forum about one woman who'd been a vegetarian for six years and then had just given up because she couldn't deal with being the only vegetarian at family events. If, I thought, someone who'd maintained a diet conducive to healing our bodies and energizing our lives for *six years* could feel such social pressure, then how much more difficult must it be for vegetarians just starting out?

The question was, of course, partly personal. I, too, knew what it was like to be the only vegetarian in my household, family, circle of friends, and place of work. I knew how it felt to be the odd one out—or thought of as just plain odd—and understood the pressure to want to fit into the meat-eating world. Why was it so hard to start and maintain something that promised so much health and wellness? How could I, let alone others, keep on this path without wandering from the road, falling off the hill, and tumbling down the mountain?

I've come to the conclusion that the reason is, in a word, *drama*. By "drama" I don't mean the challenges that life throws at us, or one's desire to act like a prima donna or diva! I'm talking about the inner battles and negativity that can all too easily surround newbie and veteran vegetarians as we try to live our lives. Although I didn't realize it at the time, my life was consumed with drama about eating. It was only when I made my way through the first thirty days, then two months, then three, then a whole year as a vegetarian that I saw that the drama and the negativity weren't necessary.

I'm now a nondramatic vegan, and in *Sister Vegetarian's 31 Days of Drama-free Living* I share my tools of success with you. This guide is a combination of my own experience and the many questions that would-be and new vegetarians have asked me about remaining on the beautiful, healthful, vegetarian journey. These questions include:

1. What makes us revert so quickly to eating meat when we're already making positive changes in our lives?
2. When we're so close to success as vegetarians, why do we act as though we have a long way to go?
3. Why does it take so long for us to become vegetarian—where we're stuck in transition mode? Why not, as the Nike slogan says, *Just Do It?*

Strong Mind

One way to maintain a vegetarian lifestyle is by having what I call a *strong mind*. With a strong mind, we can see ourselves as successful vegetarians from the beginning, acting as though we've been living a vegetarian lifestyle for years, even if we've only just begun our journey. A strong mind enables us to believe in ourselves, and see ourselves as vegetarians and not merely lapsed meat eaters. It provides what I call a "Can Do, I Can, and I Will" attitude—every day. With a strong mind we can take on the world and all it has to offer with a smile and a positive disposition because we have the proper tools. A strong mind and daily affirmations can positively reinforce "Can Do, I Can, and I Will," and lead to "I Win!" We become able to handle any situation and comments that oppose our choices. (I talk more about this subject in Day 12.)

Think about it: If we find ourselves constantly treading in a puddle of water because we can't see it, and then having to go home and dry ourselves and start again, we'd be wise to investigate why we can't see that puddle and then make sure it no longer escapes our notice. That way, not only will we see the puddle before we step in it, but we'll be able to jump over it or walk around it without starting over. A strong mind and daily positive reinforcement will enable that to happen.

I've divided this book and the positive reinforcements into thirty-one days. If you start your journey in a month with thirty or even twenty-eight days, then consider the extra days a bonus! When you've completed this book, go back to the start and follow again the progress you're making daily, weekly, monthly, and through the years. You'll see inwardly and outwardly how your confidence has increased to maintain your vegetarianism without wavering. And, guess what? You'll wake up one day and it'll dawn on you that you've been meat-free for a year! Congratulations!

I've created this book not only for individuals just starting out, but also for seasoned vegetarians who could use the inspiration and encouragement. Remember the six-year vegetarian who went back to meat? We all could use some positive reinforcement in our lives when so many voices from family, friends, and coworkers are trying to convince us that what we're doing is stupid, unnecessary, annoying, unhealthy, insulting, or obnoxious.

The tools to inspire and motivate you to never give up this vegetarian journey include:

Poems

I've included words of inspiration and motivation by up-and-coming writer Tashi S. Winston. One entitled "Encourage Yourself" sets you on your way to the start of Day 1; the other, on Day 31, and entitled "Rights of Passage Reborn," leads you to another successful month or year.

Inspirational Daily Lessons and Stories as Guides

I start off each day with a few words to inspire, motivate, and get you moving to achieve your goal(s). By using lessons and stories that I and others have learned to lead a successful vegetarian life, I hope to encourage you to believe in yourself and become who you want to be.

You Are a Shining Star

At the start of each new day, there's a space to place a star or smiley face. Vegetarianism and veganism should be fun and not stressful. Be a child again, and give yourself a star or smile to show a day completed successfully. I've also included a goals chart in Appendix III so you can give yourself more stars and smiles for personal goals reached.

Drama-free Body, Mind, and Spirit Exercises

Each day ends with exercises to inspire you even more. Sometimes they involve writing on paper or in this book; sometimes they're simply actions to repeat in order to reinforce a positive inner voice on your vegetarian journey. When we write out our goals, aspirations, and thoughts, we focus more on our words because they're in front of us. We can post them on our refrigerator, bathroom or bedroom mirrors, home or work desk, or wherever we can view them daily. Through positive actions, such as repeating mantras (as on Day 1), we mentally reinforce them and build our power to create a "can do" spirit.

Drama-free Exercise for the Body

These exercises enabled me to enjoy a fun, happy, and fulfilling exercise program before I became a vegetarian, and they were even better after I became one. Exercise is a vital component in helping us maintain a healthy, fit, and positive attitude toward life.

Drama-free Easy Recipes

Each recipe is accompanied by a small inspiring story. The recipes range in cooking time from as little as ten minutes to an hour. I've made them simple because, after a full day at the office, you want a nutritious and satisfying meal that's easy on the budget and quick to prepare so you can enjoy your evening. As part of my extra love and encouragement, I've included a bonus recipe from Chef Ricky Moore, who was the 2007 Iron Chef America Warrior in Food Network's 2007 Iron Chef America Thanksgiving Special. In addition, Sister's Weekly Meal Planner in Appendix IV will help you stay on track for a drama-free week and journey.

• • •

What makes this book different from the many vegetarian and vegan cookbooks that provide recipes for every palate, or the many books that offer self-help and inspirational wisdom? Well, *Sister Vegetarian's 31 Days of Drama-free Living* has both—and most importantly it focuses on how you can deal with the drama of when you're craving meat, or your family is sabotaging your lifestyle, or when you feel lonely and alone as the only vegetarian surrounded by meat eaters. In addition to the book, you can visit my blog At sistervegetarian.com or my Facebook or Twitter fan pages for inspirational daily quotes and stories to keep you motivated and inspired.

Finally, why Sister Vegetarian? I'm not only the younger sister of three siblings, but I consider myself a part of your family. After all, we're all sisters and brothers in this small world. Think of me as your sister in the vegetarian community—the one who offers support and guidance, with whom you can share stories and concerns and cry tears of sorrow and joy, and who'll congratulate you as you move to better health and well-being. Everyone needs help as we walk this beautiful journey. Sometimes, however, we may not have the support we want or the amount we need from blood relations. Fellow vegetarians can be your extended family, as they assist you through the storms and trials of staying away from meat. I am a part of that extended family. I am Sister Vegetarian.

Disclaimer: This book and my blog are based on my vegetarian and vegan experiences and journey as well as others' experiences. I am not a medical, nutritional, or exercise specialist; so please consult your physician before starting any vegetarian or vegan diet and exercise program.

Peace and Love,
Donna M. Beaudoin
(aka Sister Vegetarian)

encourage yourself

TASHI S. WINSTON

"Sometimes I feel like a motherless child
Sometimes I feel like a motherless child
A long way from home, a long way from home"

Mother, mother, mother hear my cry
As I scoop my life up from this lonely path
Working on my life never seemed so blurry
The vision is type hazy and I am still confused
Only to hear my voice no more
Putting up with this war alone
Still looking back on what was and used to be
Crying tears of sorrow from within
Never thought I be the one
Degree in one hand
Suffering in the other
The word HELP kills the heart and the soul
Mama where are you

Father: damn don't you remember me

Grandma I can't wait to see you

God Help me

This journey is long, but I'm standing on this victory path until the end

And walk strong

It's my time to rise and I will rise until the end is near.

Fear not, yet I have no fear.

I am fearless in my own rite and I am making it so

Bright as the sun

I'm shining . . . can you feel my heat

It's burning like fire

Like fire on a candle and I am about to blow it out

Never distant from my future for my path is already preconceived

I have faith beyond wisdom that spirals down like a stream

My head held high and walking proud for today
is the day I take back my victory.

DAY 1

victory!

As a vegetarian, you have achieved *victory* from Day 1 of starting this lifestyle change! Act as though you've been living this lifestyle for years. You're victorious the very first minute you decided to change your eating habits to a vegetarian lifestyle. You are still victorious the next one, two, or more hours, and a full day. You are victorious 24/7!

The key to becoming, maintaining, and living a vegetarian lifestyle is knowing that you have *victory* every day of your life. When you accept this mantra as your daily affirmation, you are in a win-win situation. Do you sometimes feel with family and friends as though you're in a *Star Wars* episode, when everything hangs on Darth Vader's call to his son, "Luke, come to the Dark Side." When you have confidence in yourself that you can beat the Dark Side of meat, nothing your family or friends say—whether to your face or behind your back—will compel you to return to this unhealthful lifestyle. When your mind is strong, you're

DRAMA-FREE MIND AND SPIRIT EXERCISES

1. Repeat this mantra with a smile every day, and—if possible—shout it out: *I am victorious!*

2. Write down your goals as a vegetarian. Is it to become healthier or maintain your current bill of health? When you write down your goals, you follow them through, because you've put them on paper. Post the goals where you can see them, such as your refrigerator or bathroom mirror.

3. Write down the pros and cons of following a vegetarian lifestyle. Putting them on paper (and making sure that only you see them) will make your decision easier, because you'll realize that the pros always outweigh the cons.

4. Surround yourself with a positive support group—such as the many vegetarian forums, websites, blogs, and community groups.

5. Remember: Positive reinforcement supports your personal *victory!*

better able to deal with and conquer any situation.

You have a strong mind. So I want you to say to yourself that you are victorious today and every day. Say it now: *I am victorious!* Repeat it louder: *I am victorious!* Say it again and again: *I am victorious! I am victorious!*

It feels good, doesn't it? Your mind and body are rejuvenated; your inner spirit is renewed. You find yourself saying, *Huh! I got this. I am victorious every day of my life on this vegetarian journey!*

Repeat this mantra every day and you'll feel a positive change. You won't want to turn back to meat if you reinforce your success within your mind. You don't want to let yourself down. When you build confidence in yourself, you have the self-assurance to conquer all things. You develop a can-do attitude and believe in yourself. You need to give yourself a chance to enable that. *I am victorious!*

Do you believe it now? Yes, you do! Why? Because, in adopting a vegetarian lifestyle, you've made a conscious decision not only to take back your health, but, if you're already healthy, to provide a wall of defense and protection against the cold, the flu, cancer, heart disease, diabetes, and other illnesses. I can't, of course, guarantee that you won't ever get sick, but I *can* tell you that you've lessened your chances for contracting these illnesses or diseases. Your body is stronger and able to fight *for* you rather than against you. You can heal your body through vegetarianism and keep it healthy.

As I mentioned in the introduction, I know this from personal experience. I was hospitalized four times within a ten-year period for acute stomach pain that my physicians were at a loss to diagnose. I was also constantly sick with bacterial and viral infections. After a year of living a vegetarian lifestyle, the stomach pains had vanished. For over a year, I was virus- and flu-free—without taking any shots.

Hippocrates, the Father of Modern Medicine, is reputed to have said, "Let your food be your medicine, and your medicine your food." I would agree. As my vegetarian food healed me, I became healthier and stronger mentally, physically, and spiritually. I was getting up at five o'clock in the morning and riding

DRAMA-FREE EXERCISE FOR THE BODY

Victory starts with you. Begin an exercise program at a time of day that will enable you to maintain it on a daily basis. Studies have shown that we stay on an exercise program not by joining a gym but by doing something we love at a time of the day when we know we have the energy and time to stick with an exercise program. If you're an early riser, fit it in at five a.m. before you get ready for work. Do you prefer to sleep late? Then six or eight p.m. may be better for you. Select the time that fits into your busy schedule as a working person, single parent, entrepreneur, caregiver, etc. Time for yourself is paramount if you want to maintain a drama-free life. What is your established exercise time?

a stationary bike for an hour, five days a week. I practiced yoga, ran long-distance races, and hiked and backpacked on the weekends. I went from a size fourteen to a size four in less than a year. I had more energy at age forty-three than when I was in my twenties and thirties. I felt and still feel more alive!

Do you believe in yourself? Adopt a can-do attitude. You *can*! You *will*! You are *victorious*!

victory! i am alive and well curried raw beet greens salad

VEGAN

My great-grandmother, Otis Mae Robinson, was born and raised in Alabama before she moved to California in the 1930s. She was proud of her Southern upbringing and her commitment to good nutrition. She ate beets weekly, if not more often, and regularly ate raw salads made of beet greens. My mother introduced me to beets as a toddler, and I've loved them ever since. It's a myth that children hate vegetables; they'll eat whatever you put in front of them. They develop their dislike of foods from the comments that parents make at the dinner table. Children do listen!

Let's be positive examples to our children, nieces, nephews, and grandchildren, through making wise choices and eating healthfully. Let's start with this beautiful, purplish vegetable that's packed with nutrients that halt the body's aging process. Most vitally, it protects us from colon cancer. Whether you eat the buttery- and sweet-tasting beet by itself or in combination with the slightly salty green leaves and stems, the beet acts as a natural detoxifier and prevents cardiovascular disease. I eat both root and stems every week to keep my colon free from toxins. It's a pretty package that Mother Earth gives to us to renew, grow, and energize our healthy cells.

I eat beets both raw and cooked in salads, Indian lentil stews, with pasta, and mixed with beans and legumes. Besides having more vitamins, antioxidants, and cancer-fighting nutrients than common lettuce, beet greens have many flavors packed into their leaves.

I'm incredibly proud of the contribution that the collard greens, mustard greens, turnip greens, beet greens, kale, and Swiss chard of my Southern and African-American heritages have made to our national cuisine. These beautiful vegetables have been called "slave greens," "soul food," "black food," and now "live" or "raw greens"—a testimony to their complicated journey through the American psyche. I didn't always consider them so highly. Even though I grew up eating these foods, during college in New England and after graduation I mixed more with students from non-Southern states and fell into the trap of thinking that eating greens was too Southern—by which I mean that I believed them to be unsophisticated and rustic.

Nonetheless, in more ways than one, you can't forget your roots; you always come back home. I finally returned to my senses and whence I came—not geographically, but to the culinary ways of my parents, grandparents, great-grandparents, and assorted aunts, uncles, cousins, and ancestors in Alabama, Georgia, and South Carolina—who understood the value and importance of the bounty that Mother Earth provides. In both a literal and metaphorical sense, the collards, mustards, turnips, beets, and kale kept my family going through the years of slavery and Jim Crow. They were the ground that fed and nurtured us, and the way we asserted our identity, individuality, and racial pride. They made sure we didn't get sick, and that we stayed strong both physically and mentally.

Now my roots are, quite literally, a part of me: whether in hearty stews, delicious side dishes, or refreshing salads. It's almost like they're saying: "We welcome you back with love, prodigal daughter. You were never gone from us."

Through the decades, traditional Southern and African-American recipes have seasoned and simmered the roots in water. However, cooking methods have emerged that provide a whole new world of eating your greens. Not only are they displayed on Food Network shows such as Bobby Flay's and Rachel Ray's, but they're taught in culinary schools. You can even find them in raw food restaurants from New York to Los Angeles and on the menu of four- and five-starred restaurants. The humble greens have arrived!

As you'll see throughout this book, I like to eat different salads topped with beets, lentils, black beans, eggplant, or more bounty from Mother Earth. I enjoy collard wraps for lunch stuffed with these greens, as opposed to lettuce. Not only do I find them tastier, but they serve to connect me with my grandparents' and great-grandparents' generation.

These leafy greens are full of more nutrients than the lettuce that populates the Standard American Diet (SAD). Swiss chard has been shown to possess antioxidant and anti-inflammatory properties and to assist in fighting cancer. High in calcium, potassium, iron, protein, and fiber, it supports healthy bones and is an excellent source for vitamins K, A, C, E, and B$_6$. Turnip greens have a slightly bitter taste, with a hint of white pepper, and are beneficial in colon health, detoxification, and in aiding digestion. They are powerful antioxidants and anti-inflammatories, and provide minerals such as calcium, niacin, potassium, and iron. In addition to being rich with protein and fiber, turnip greens are sources of vitamins K, A, C, E, B_1, B_2, and B_5.

Collard greens have a buttery and slightly sweet taste. They provide assistance in fighting cancer, detoxifying the body, aiding digestion and cardiovascular health, and easing menopausal symptoms. They are excellent sources of vitamins K, A, C, E, B_2, B_5, and B_6, and are filled with calcium, potassium, iron, protein, and fiber. Beet greens are bitter, and contain many of the same properties as the other greens. They are also good sources of vitamin C and folate. Kale, which is sweet and crisp in taste, is also useful in treating the above conditions, and can also protect your eyes against cataracts.

The above positive qualities found in these greens are why I don't use the common lettuce varieties such as iceberg, romaine, butter, mesclun, oak leaf, etc. I like to go above and beyond and raise the bar for a salad—one that's not only full of flavor but packed with antioxidants, cancer-fighting properties, and high in vitamins, cardiovascular protection, lung health, and loads of calcium to promote strong bones.

For this recipe, I used the entire beet—root, greens, and stems—and did so without peeling the root, since the skin also contains nutrients. In decades past, African Americans and Eastern Europeans often ate entire beets (greens, roots, and stems) for strength, health, and vitality. We rarely suffered from cardiovascular diseases, diabetes, or cancer problems in such numbers until we introduced ourselves to the SAD of processed foods. Mother Earth provides it all! Don't eat SAD iceberg, romaine, and other common lettuces. Eat your greens!

Preparation and Cooking Time: 20 minutes
Serving: 1

Ingredients

Curried Raw Beet Greens Salad

4 cups noncooked beet greens, washed. Roughly cut with about four inches of the stem left on. Stem is cut in half and added to salad.

1/2 cup yellow onions, sliced

1 clove medium garlic, minced

Marinade

1/8 cup extra virgin olive oil

1/8 cup organic maple syrup

1/8 cup organic raw apple cider vinegar

1/8 tsp ground black pepper

1 tsp ground curry

1 tsp cumin

1 tsp ground coriander

1/2 tsp turmeric

Optional: For a lacto-vegetarian version of the salad, add a slice or two of fresh mozzarella cheese cut in half-inch slices, and place on top.

Optional: Serve crusty Italian bread, warmed, and drizzled with olive oil.

Oven Grilled Beets

Olive oil

1 small beet, washed and sliced in half- to one-inch rounds with the skin left on

Smoked paprika

Ground chipotle pepper

Vegan liquid smoke

Directions
Oven Grilled Beets Preparation

1. Preheat oven to broil.
2. Lightly coat an oven pan with olive oil.
3. Add sliced beets to pan.
4. Sprinkle lightly smoked paprika and ground chipotle. Add a few drops of vegan liquid smoke.
5. Place in oven on broil. Broil four to five minutes on each side until just tender, but not fully tender. Beets should have a crunch.

Curried Raw Beet Greens Salad Preparation

1. As beets broil in oven, combine beet greens with onions and garlic in a bowl. Mix with hands or tongs. I tend to mix with my (well-washed) hands, which do the job better than tongs or a spoon, and at the same time I'm giving my positive energy and love to the meal preparation.
2. Combine salad marinade in a separate bowl or salad bottle. Mix with fork or shake bottle.
3. Add marinade to bowl of greens mixture, and mix with hands.
4. Set aside for five minutes to marinate (beet greens will shrink).

Combine All

1. When beets are done in the oven, add to the marinated salad and toss with tongs or your hands.
2. Serve on a beautiful plate or pasta bowl. Pasta bowls are not just for pasta. I love them for serving stews, soups, and salads because they are wide like a plate, but hold salads well inside.

DAY 2

goals can help you maintain a vegetarian lifestyle

If you reach for something when you're not ready, then you have a greater chance of failing—hence the reason why so many vegetarians start out on this wonderful journey and don't reach their goal. You'll be much more likely to succeed if you set small targets and take small steps that allow you to monitor your progress, reward your accomplishments, and make adjustments as necessary. When you reach one goal, set another. A plan like this enables you to stay on the vegetarian path, because you're able to see your growth and advancement daily, rather than concentrating on the end result, which may be weeks, months, or a year away. This is hard. We're a society that gets a high off instant gratification. If we can't see some type of progress right away, we tend to give up.

The truth is, we're already succeeding on our path as vegetarians, but we overlook the little joys, achievements, and accomplishments we experience along the way because we're too focused on the result. In fact, we don't realize that the best moments of the journey are those small steps, not the end. By being on the path, we've *already* succeeded.

My first goal on my vegetarian journey was to start to become healthy by instituting a vegetarian diet in my life. I didn't know what my next goal would be. I thought that if I could complete a full week as a vegetarian, without being sidetracked, then the first of many goals in living a golden, healthy life would have been reached. Once I met my first goal of completing a full week, I made another goal: to go a full thirty days. That then became two months, then three, and then six.

During this time, I began to drop the weight I'd gained in three-and-a-half years. So, I decided to add another goal: to lose one to two pounds a week. Once I'd completed six months as a vegetarian, I thought to myself: "Donna, do you want your goal to stay on a monthly or yearly basis?" I concluded that I'd achieved so much by setting monthly goals—monitoring my progress and seeing results—that I should continue this way. Nonetheless, I added yet another goal: of getting back in shape with a consistent program at the time of day I knew least likely to provide me with excuses for not exercising.

By working in small steps, I found myself able to continue to add goals, but not to feel overwhelmed by the process. With my exercise program, for instance, I allotted periods in the morning before work, because that time worked best for me. I started with thirty minutes of exercise. Within a few weeks, I was working out for a full hour—mainly because I had more energy and enthusiasm. Indeed, I found myself wanting to hike more, camp, and learn how to backpack. I

DRAMA-FREE MIND AND SPIRIT EXERCISES

1. Write out your goals on a chart. Place goals in one column, the start date of the goal in the second, and the completion date of the goal in the third. The fourth column is your reward. When you achieve it, be a kid again and have fun. Purchase some sticky stars and put one next to the goal. Or just buy crayons and draw stars in different colors.

2. Appendix III has a sample Goals Chart. Tear it out or photocopy it and use it to set goals for a successful vegetarian journey.

3. Don't forget to place a star or smiley face at the top of each Daily Motivation in the space provided called "Day Completed _____." This star is your motivation and inspiration for each day completed on your vegetarian journey. When you finish, this will be your book of accomplishments. Show everyone, and refer to it yourself for continued motivation. Yes, you can do it!

wrote down these additional goals and successfully reached them in small steps.

After a year, I decided to run again after a ten-year hiatus from running, where I only averaged three to eight miles at the most. Once again, I began with small steps. I consulted books and the Internet and found a program that I thought would work for me. Only ten weeks into my program, I came in fourth in my age group in a 5K (3.1 mile) race. A month later, I ran a ten-mile race, and two weeks after that I ran a half marathon (13.1 miles), which I'll describe in more detail later in the book. As you can imagine, this exercise regimen contributed to further weight loss, so that I went from a size fourteen to four in less than a year. None of these steps required great leaps of willpower or discipline. In fact, the new goals I set for myself emerged from my enthusiasm and desire to do more. All I did was to set goals to eat healthful, whole foods as a vegetarian and leave time for daily exercise.

So, take small steps. Small steps lead to big accomplishments. There's no need to be overwhelmed or force yourself to be like someone else. Write down your goals for you and you only. Don't hitch a ride on someone else's cloud. It's all about you and no one else.

DRAMA-FREE EXERCISE FOR THE BODY

Eating healthfully is important, but so is exercise. One without the other is like a pot without a stove to cook on. Exercise and healthful vegetarian eating go hand-in-hand for prolonged, positive health. Set an exercise goal. Stick to small goals that lead to more daily exercise. For example, start by walking fifteen minutes a day. By the second or third week, increase the time to thirty minutes, then forty-five minutes, then one hour—if that is your goal. Carving out time can initially be hard; but small steps and small goals make it easier.

DRAMA-FREE EASY RECIPE

just like grandma vegan cinnamon-raisin wheat bread

VEGAN

Setting goals includes planning lunch and dinner. Plan your lunch meals for the week, with homemade bread made on the weekend.

My great-grandmother, Otis Mae Robinson, and her daughter believed in goals both for themselves and their community in a time of a national crisis. My mother told me that during World War II, my grandmother and great-grandmother would help people in their San Francisco neighborhood supplement their food rations by baking bread. Otis Mae would eventually open a restaurant called The Virginia Diner in Vallejo, California. The specialty of the diner was bean stews such as chili, with homemade bread as an accompaniment. I not only find homemade bread delicious and nutritious, but it brings up memories of the snow days of my New Jersey childhood, when my mother would bake bread. Remembering the smell of my own childhood allows me to visualize what my great-grandmother and grandmother's home in San Francisco must have been like as they baked bread for the community.

Home-baked bread not only warms the stomach, the hearth, and the community, but it delivers the love we pour into the kneading of the dough. It brings families and people together to "break bread," as my childhood minister would say. Such an outpouring of love reminds us of generations before us who gave of themselves and shared with their neighbors during a time when they had little to spare and may have been on rations themselves.

Aside from the connections we can build with our past and the people around us, homemade bread provides more nutrients and flavor. You can add or take away extra ingredients—such as the fruit—should you just want basic bread. You can share this quick, "no-knead" recipe with neighbors, family, and friends. Make two, three, four, or ten for your community. It's quick and vegan!

Cooking Time: 1 hour
Servings: 1 loaf baked in an approximately
8 1/2-inch x 4 1/2-inch bread pan

Ingredients

1/4 cup vegetable oil

3 cups wheat flour

Vegetable oil to lightly coat baking pan and plastic cover for bread as it rises

1 cup lukewarm water

1/4 cup rice milk (oat milk, soymilk, almond milk, or coconut milk can be substituted)

1 1/2 oz package of active yeast (equivalent to 2 1/4 tsp yeast)

3 tbsp organic brown sugar

1 tbsp cinnamon

1/2 cup chopped fresh orange. Peel skin, deseed, and chop.

1 cup raisins

Directions

1. Grease the bread pan with vegetable oil.
2. Pour the wheat flour in bowl. Make a well in the center of the flour and add the oil, water, and milk ingredients. Add the remaining ingredients and stir with a wooden spoon until just mixed. Then use your hands of love and positive energy to continue to mix the ingredients until all are fully mixed. Your hands when mixing will simulate a slight kneading motion in the bowl, but this should only take two to three minutes.
3. Scoop the bread mixture with your hands into the oiled bread pan.
4. Cover the pan with lightly greased plastic or wax paper, and let it rise for ninety minutes on your counter.
5. Preheat oven to 350 degrees F.

6. Place the uncovered bread in the oven, and bake for fifty to sixty minutes.

7. Insert a knife to determine if the bread is done. The bread is done if the knife comes out clean.

8. Cool the bread completely before slicing it. I slice the bread and store it in a freezer bag in my refrigerator. It can be reheated when used.

Note: You can add all or part of the fruit as indicated or leave out the fruit for a basic wheat bread. The baking time will shorten by ten to fifteen minutes, or until done.

DAY 3

tired of being sick and tired (my story)

As I wrote in the introduction, I used to feel unwell a lot. I couldn't work out why I was gaining weight or why I kept on getting stomach pains and colds and viruses. What was happening to my body? The physicians couldn't find an answer. I had constant stomach pains; and, although I exercised, I still gained weight.

I still had an appetite. I ate lots of meat, with few to no vegetables accompanying the dishes. I blamed my problems on getting older (I'd just turned forty). What I didn't grasp was that meat was the source of all the problems I was experiencing. I wasn't looking at the full picture of my life, but trying to make excuses for myself and blame something else.

Not only had my weight increased from 110 to 148 lbs., and no longer a size four but a twelve, bordering on fourteen, but my hips had expanded from thirty-five inches to forty-two and my waist from twenty-five inches to thirty-one. My face had become swollen because of the toxicity that had built up in my colon from eating meat and few vegetables.

Curiously enough, I considered myself a health-conscious person. After all, I exercised for an hour each day and hiked on weekends. I ate more poultry than red meat. I cooked at home and didn't eat in restaurants much, and in fast-food joints infrequently. As a teenager I'd preferred oven-baked and oven-fried foods to deep-fried meals. I'd also loved my vegetables. However, as I'd grown older, they'd disappeared from my plate as meat had taken up more and more space. I'd even started to eat BBQ ribs, as I'd embraced my new home of North Carolina. I'd married a meat lover, which I used as another excuse not only to avoid becoming a vegetarian, but transitioning back to meat eating when I became one. Why should I bother cooking two meals—one for him and one for me?—I asked myself.

It felt as hard to give up chicken as if I were on drugs. Meat eating was woven into every part of my day. After my hikes, I'd come back and eat a heavy, meat-based meal. While watching my beloved New York Yankees baseball team on TV, I'd consume a huge New York–style sandwich (with half a pound of meat) and drink beer. I love football almost as much as baseball, and so this kind of sport-bingeing would be a year-round activity.

One day, I asked a question dreaded by every husband: "Do I look fat?"

"No, baby," he responded, tactfully. "You look good. I like your butt."

I can't blame him—what man isn't a butt man?—and in a funny way I was pleased. Maybe that extra thirty-eight pounds *did* make me look good. But then I had to remember that I was only five-foot-two inches tall. I wasn't experiencing a bowel movement for three or four days at a time. I'd had to give away my favorite clothes because I couldn't fit into them anymore. Simply climbing a flight of stairs would leave me out of breath, and when I hiked I found it hard to keep up with the others without huffing and puffing and having back pains. Heart disease runs on both sides of my family; consequently, when I felt heart palpitations and shortness of breath, I began to think I was showing signs of heart disease. (Thankfully, visits to my physician proved me wrong.)

I decided to find out the source of the problem. I visited my ob-gyn, who conducted an ultrasound to make sure my pelvic discomfort wasn't caused by cysts. Although the physician commented on my weight gain, she made no suggestions when the tests came back clear. I went to my internist, who performed X-rays and a colonoscopy, since my uncles had died of colon and stomach cancer. The tests were all clear. I told the internist that I'd never weighed as much and that I was getting heavier, but he appeared to ignore the implications. "Well, the tests came back fine," he said. "So maybe it's just stress."

For a month after the colonoscopy, I felt a little better. My bowel movements increased and, while I didn't lose weight, at least I didn't gain any. Six months after the colonoscopy, however, I caught a bad cold and stomach infection that forced me to stay away from work for a couple of days. While I was home, I prayed to God to show me what to do to get healthy. The message came through loud and clear. All my ailments were the result of toxicity in my colon, and a vegetarian diet would clean up my colon naturally. It was the last week of February.

I started eating a vegetarian diet and performed a natural colon cleansing. By the end of the following month I'd lost eight pounds. Two weeks later, I'd lost another eight. I no longer felt pain in my shoulders, pelvis, stomach, or legs. I could walk upstairs and hike without being out of breath, and the backaches stopped. My bowel movements became regular, daily occurrences, which doctors consider a basic requirement for health.

You would think that, having asked God for guidance a few months previously, I would have learned my lesson. But we want to believe that our minds are strong enough to fight the temptations of a meat-based diet. In the last week in May, my husband and I went camping and hiking, to climb a couple of summits in the Blue Ridge Mountains. I decided

DRAMA-FREE MIND AND SPIRIT EXERCISES

1. Let's think for ourselves, and take back our health. Question your physicians, and ask them how you can reduce the number of medications you take.
2. Plan "No Excuse Meals." Use the recipes in this book. Go to your local library to try out vegetarian cookbooks before purchasing them for your home collection. When you own a library of great vegetarian recipes from quick meals to more elaborate ones for family gatherings, you'll have no excuse for not finding something to eat.
3. If you work, compile recipes of quick vegetarian meals that take thirty minutes or less to make.
4. Prepare stews, soups, or larger meals on Saturdays and Sundays. Freeze the leftovers, and reheat them during the week after work for a quick meal.
5. See Appendix II for further resources. When we educate ourselves, we have choices; we're more aware and take our lives into our own hands. We become the catalyst for change rather than waiting for someone else to tell us what to do, which may not be right for us. As James Colquhoun, the producer and director of the documentary *Food Matters,* says, "It's about education, not medication."

to eat meat on the trip because I thought that with all the hiking I'd be doing, I'd need to keep my strength up. And then I didn't stop eating meat for five months! Sure enough, my face began to swell and my bowel movements started to decrease. I put on four pounds.

On October 22, 2009, I finally returned to vegetarianism—I believe for life. In so doing, I've discovered a new world of flavors and recipes. I'm now stronger, fitter, and more energetic in my midforties than I've been for many years. Even though I work in a medical facility and am surrounded by people who have colds, flus, and viruses of varying kinds, I've remained flu-free since becoming a vegetarian. My aches and pains and illnesses have vanished. As my great-grandmother believed, nature has cures for colds and flus—and she should know. She lived to be a vivacious, active centenarian, until she departed this earth in 1993, and incorporated healthful vegetarian meals into her diet.

While I started as a lacto-ovo vegetarian, I've now become a vegan. You may want to remain an ovo-, lacto-, or lacto-ovo vegetarian. Your goal may be to transition to veganism, or you may start out as a vegan. Whatever your goal may be, however, be proud of whatever path you choose. Take back your health, and make a decision to live healthily on a daily basis.

DRAMA-FREE EXERCISES FOR THE BODY

Start an exercise program slowly and build up to a goal. Set small goals to maintain your program.

DRAMA-FREE EASY RECIPE

sick no more curried split-pea soup with sweet potatoes and mustard greens

VEGAN

Besides eating healthful, whole foods, I add curry to many of my meals. In addition to being a staple spice in Indian food, curry can be found in many Asian, Caribbean, and Mexican cuisines. Curry is comprised of four main ingredients—coriander, cumin, fenugreek, and turmeric—with the addition of other spices depending on the type you use. These spices provide protection against colds, and their properties can heal you if you have a cold or the flu by giving a boost to your immune system. Cumin can also open your nasal passages if you feel stuffed up or suffer from asthma. The mustard greens used in this recipe also help you breathe more easily if you're suffering from a cold or the flu, or have asthma. An excellent source of vitamins K, A, C, E, and B_6, as well as calcium, protein, and fiber, mustard greens have been known to ease the symptoms of menopause, increase mental efficiency and awareness, and offer protection against rheumatoid arthritis.

Cooking Time: approximately 1 hour
Servings: 4–6

Ingredients

2 tbsp extra virgin olive oil

1 medium jalapeño chili pepper, minced (I left my seeds and veins in for more heat, but feel free to deseed and de-vein for less heat).

1 medium onion, chopped

2 tbsp ground curry

2 tsp ground cumin

1 tsp ground ginger

4 garlic cloves, minced

1 16-oz. bag of dried split peas (any color, cleaned and soaked overnight according to bag instructions)

8 cups water

2 medium sweet potatoes (cleaned and skin left on for more nutrients), cut into one-inch cubes

1 vegan vegetable bouillon cube

4 cups coarsely chopped mustard greens

Garlic salt to taste

Ground black pepper to taste

Garnish: homemade Italian croutons (Italian bread, extra virgin olive oil, and dry Italian seasonings)

Directions

1. Add 2 tbsp olive oil to a large pot.
2. Sauté the jalapeño pepper, onions, curry, cumin, ginger, and garlic.
3. Add the split peas and sauté for two minutes.
4. Add the water, sweet potatoes, and bouillon cube.
5. Boil then turn down heat to simmer, forty-five to fifty minutes.

6. Add mustard greens to pot, and simmer for five minutes. Season with salt and pepper to taste. Serve in individual bowls.
7. Garnish: Toast Italian bread in the broiler with a sprinkle of dry Italian seasonings and extra virgin olive oil. Cut the bread in cubes and sprinkle on top of the soup. Use garlic salt and pepper to taste.

DAY 4

become an activist for change by talking to your local grocery store

My local grocery store listens to me. Yes, *me*! An average, middle-class, middle-aged, working woman. I never saw myself as an activist or catalyst for change in my neighborhood. But, in this case, I felt it was important to speak up for what I believed in. I wanted to see fresher and more organic produce and products at the store, not just to support my vegetarian lifestyle within my budget but also to help other people in my community lead healthier lives. I wanted to institute the means by which patrons wouldn't need to travel across town to shop for healthier produce and products.

I live in an area where incomes range from impoverished to middle

DRAMA-FREE MIND AND SPIRIT EXERCISES

1. Make a list of things you like and don't like about your shopping experience at your local grocery store. On that list, pinpoint how you want the store to change, add things, or keep the same. Remember, grocery stores should cater to all, not just those who eat meat or junk food.
2. If you don't have a computer to access the grocery store's website, use your local library's free computers or call the toll-free phone number. If the store doesn't have a website or phone number, then ask to speak to the manager.
3. Give feedback every time you shop at your grocery store—even if you just run in for one item. The more the store hears from you, the faster the change will come, because they'll see how serious and committed you are to making a positive change in your neighborhood.
4. Hold the store accountable. If after a month you don't see at least one change from your feedback, indicate how surprised you are that the status quo remains. Let the store know you're watching and taking note. The corporate and local offices will realize that you're serious. You'll then see changes being made.
5. Congratulations! You've made a change in your local grocery store. Continue to give feedback. See other changes taking place. You're now an activist for positive change in your local store. You may even have an effect on other stores in similar neighborhoods. I'm proud of you!

class; usually, these areas are the last to see healthier products in the stores. I got tired of going to the grocery store near where I worked, which was located in an affluent community where people could purchase organic, nongenetically modified, and vegetarian produce and products. I felt my local grocery store should provide the same to its own community. Just because one area is affluent doesn't mean that a less wealthy area isn't filled with individuals who have the same desire to buy quality fresh, vegetarian, organic, and nongenetically modified fare.

The store cashiers kept encouraging patrons to visit their store's website or call the toll-free number after their shopping experience to give feedback. The store even offered an opportunity to win free groceries as an incentive. Each week after a trip to the grocery store, I'd leave comments on the website. I still do, to show them that I and others are continuing to pay attention and are concerned about the food available in our community. Though I've yet to win free groceries, I have changed the store, and that makes me feel a winner!

DRAMA-FREE EXERCISE FOR THE BODY

Walking relaxes, reduces stress, and keeps the mind, body, and spirit in tip-top shape. Walk to the grocery store, the post office, and work. Walk at lunchtime. Walk for exercise. Walk for your health.

I make sure to say "thank you" for positive changes and to show someone is watching. For instance, I noticed that the store had introduced organic apples, and expressed my appreciation on the website. Within a couple of weeks, a special section had been designed for organic produce. The area was small, but it was a step in the right direction. It felt good to know I was being heard and taken seriously by the store's corporate office and the local management.

If your local grocery stores do not have the produce and products you need to lead a healthful vegetarian lifestyle, don't give up. Take action. Become the active force to make a change for you and your community. These stores will never improve if you don't speak up. Speak up once, twice, three times, and more until they make a change.

Don't be afraid. If you speak up, others will be encouraged to follow suit, and your voice will be heard. If you remain silent, however, the stores will continue to supply products based on market research that doesn't apply to you, and conclude that you're okay with the status quo.

However, if you feel your grocery store isn't meeting your needs, and that it should provide reasonably priced, quality items for you and others to live healthy lives in your neighborhood, then you need to say: "I want to make a change. Let me show you how."

Sitting at home complaining about things doesn't bring about change. The women and men who fought for civil rights and women's rights from the 1950s to the 1970s decided to act. If Gloria Steinem, Abbie Hoffman, Rosa Parks, Kwame Ture (aka Stokely Carmichael), Martin Luther King, Jr., Malcolm X, Fannie Lou Hamer, and many others hadn't stood up for what they believed in and instigated change, we wouldn't have the opportunities we have today.

DRAMA-FREE EASY RECIPE

nathaniel gaskins' sixteen bean soup

VEGAN

I recently discovered that my great-great-grandfather, Nathaniel Gaskins, was a soldier during the Civil War. As a former slave, he stood up for what he believed in by joining the Union Army to fight for a country that mistreated him. He knew he might be able to help make a difference and bring about positive changes. Soldiers during the Civil War ate what they could (which wasn't much) and relied on meals of various dry-bean soups. I love bean soups, and when I make my many versions of bean soups—especially this sixteen dry-bean version—I think of how my great-great-grandfather may have eaten a similar version while fighting for our freedom and rights.

Every grocery store carries dried sixteen- or thirteen-bean mixtures: either version can be used, or you can purchase the beans in bulk at a store. Make sure the dry-bean bag indicates only beans, since many brands now mix the beans with meat and spices.

Cooking Time: approximately 1 hour
Servings: 4–6

Ingredients

1 16-oz. pkg. 16 dry-beans soup mix (only beans, no added seasonings in package)

8 cups of water

1 vegan vegetable bouillon cube

2 15 1/2 oz. cans diced, roasted garlic tomatoes

2 cups fresh mustard greens, roughly chopped (use everything: leaves and stems)

1 10-oz. package of frozen, sliced carrots

1 large onion, chopped

2 tsp ground cumin

2 tsp ground curry

1 tsp ground ginger

4 cloves garlic, minced

3–4 pieces of chipotle peppers in adobo sauce, chopped

2 cups fresh turnip greens, roughly chopped (use everything: leaves and stems)

Directions

1. Clean and soak dry beans according to package instructions.
2. Add water and bouillon cube to a large pot. Boil until bouillon cube is dissolved in water. Stir.

3. Add all remaining ingredients (including cleaned and soaked beans) except greens.
4. Boil. Lower the heat to simmer.
5. Simmer for one hour.
6. Add greens to pot for five minutes.
7. Remove from heat and serve.

DAY 5 COMPLETED: _____

take a step of faith

You've already made the first step toward being a vegetarian. Reward yourself. You're on your way. Now take another step. Being a vegetarian involves faith: inner faith when no one else around you at home, at work, or in your circle of friends is a vegetarian; faith, when you're constantly asked why you chose this lifestyle. "How can you give up meat?" And, tiresomely and ubiquitously: "Where does your protein come from?" You'll also be accused by family members of turning your back on how you were raised, as if their way of eating is no longer good enough for you.

Faith will carry you through the good times, the bad times, and answering those redundant questions of *why . . . why . . . why.* Of course, some people are genuinely curious and their inquiries will be worth answering. You may even touch someone's heart and mind in the process, and get them thinking of becoming a vegetarian. But other ques-

DRAMA-FREE MIND AND SPIRIT EXERCISES

1. Build your faith. Find a mantra: whether in this book, from your favorite author, or religious scripture, and make it your daily mantra. Meditate on the statement daily until you memorize it. Believe in it. Make it your victory song.
2. When you encounter a setback, repeat your mantra and jump back on track.
3. Don't be hard on yourself. Accept that you can make mistakes, and that you're human. Accept that the beauty of another day is that you can change what you did the day before, and start over again as a new person.

DRAMA-FREE EXERCISE FOR THE BODY

Walk or run with a group for motivation. Join a beginner's women or co ed walking/running program in your area. Log on to meetup.com for a list of local groups.

tions will merely be attempts by self-centered people to test you and sabotage your new journey. Faith enables you to calmly hold your ground, and refrain from wringing their necks!

Faith will also pull you up and get you back on the right track if you should falter and eat those hot chicken wings. You'll realize that you're human and can make mistakes. You'll accept your faults and not linger on the setbacks. You'll get yourself right back up, and on the path to vegetarianism because you know that the journey is not over. You will not be defeated. You will keep on moving forward to heal your body, to preserve the environment, and support animal welfare. Faith gives you the strength to move mountains, climb hills, and wake up in the morning knowing that you want to follow your vegetarian lifestyle.

If your faith isn't strong enough to sustain you through the vegetarian journey, then put on your shield of strength and increase it. Be a Wonder Woman or a Superman, and allow your shield to deflect the negativity thrown at you. Use daily mantras and meditations to encourage, motivate, and inspire you. When you believe in yourself, your faith increases. When faith increases, you know that anything is possible, if you believe in yourself. Believe that you can, and you will. Have faith and you will go far on this vegetarian journey. Prove it to yourself!

vegan-style huevos rancheros (scrambled tofu topped with cuban aioli spicy avocado sauce)

VEGAN

Every day, farmers take a step in faith. They have faith that the seeds they sow will become healthful, abundant vegetables in time. I am in awe of farmers for their hard and meaningful work.

Huevos rancheros (*huevos* means eggs, and *rancheros* means ranch style) is a Mexican dish that, at one time, farm workers ate for breakfast to fuel them until dinner. Actually, this dish can be eaten any time of day. I prefer it as a quick-to-prepare, light dinner. There are many variations to huevos rancheros. In my version, I use tofu instead of eggs. You can always add or take away ingredients—nonetheless, what make huevos rancheros the dish it is are the eggs or egg substitutes, beans, tomatoes, or salsa sauce as traditionally used, and avocados.

Ingredients

Scrambled Tofu

1 14-oz. package of firm tofu, drained

2 tbsp olive oil

1/4 cup chopped onions

1/2 small jalapeño pepper (deveined, deseeded, and diced)

1/4 cup chopped green peppers

1/2 tsp turmeric

1/2 tsp cumin

2 tbsp nutritional yeast

Garlic salt and black pepper to taste

Bean and Tomato Sauce

1/2 cup onion, minced

3 medium cloves garlic, chopped

1 tbsp cilantro leaves, minced

1 tsp ground cumin

1/4 tsp ground chipotle pepper

2 tbsp extra virgin olive oil to sauté sauce and lightly coat egg-cooking pan

1 cup diced roasted-garlic canned tomatoes, undrained

1 cup of canned black beans, drained

1/8 cup fresh chopped mustard greens

1 cup shredded fresh collard greens, turnip greens, or mustard greens

Cuban Aioli Sauce (recipe below)

Cuban Aioli Sauce

Aioli originated in Provençal (France) as a dip, sandwich spread, or accompaniment to grilled meats or vegetables. Cooking regions adapted aioli to make it their own, such as this Cuban version I made by reinventing aioli using a southern ingredient (mustard greens). The main ingredient in aioli is mayonnaise (I use vegan mayonnaise). However, you can create your own versions from this main ingredient.

Aioli Sauce Ingredients

1 Hass avocado, halved, pitted, and peeled

1/4 cup vegan mayonnaise

1 tbsp lemon juice

4 medium garlic cloves, peeled

1–2 chipotle pepper halves in adobo sauce, depending on how hot you prefer the sauce

1/2 cup mustard greens leaves

1/2 tsp sea salt

1/2 tsp vegan liquid smoke

Aioli Sauce Directions

Mix all ingredients above in a food processor. Store in an airtight container or a glass jar. It keeps in the refrigerator for five to seven days.

Vegan Style Huevos Rancheros Directions

1. Prepare Mexican aioli sauce and set aside.
2. In a pan, sauté onion, garlic, cilantro, cumin, and ground chipotle in 2 tbsp olive oil for one to two minutes.
3. Add diced tomatoes, 1/8 cup mustard greens, and black beans. Cook on low, until heated throughout. Set aside.
4. In the meantime, crumble tofu in a pan lightly oiled with olive oil. Add onions, jalapeño pepper, and green peppers to the tofu and sauté on medium heat for three minutes. Add turmeric, cumin, and nutritional yeast. Cook for another five minutes until fluffy. Season with garlic salt and pepper to taste.

5. Plate bean, tomato, and spice mixture on top of a bed of 1 cup of shredded greens of your choice. Place scrambled tofu on top. Place a dollop (as desired) of Mexican aioli sauce on top of tofu and/or on side of plate for additional sauce. An alternative to the aioli sauce is half a chopped avocado placed on top of scrambled tofu.

6. Serve.

DAY 6

we come in all sizes

There's a misconception that all vegetarians, especially vegans, are extremely thin. This myth seems to be held by nonvegetarians, newbie vegetarians, and (to my surprise) some veterans who want to adopt a vegan lifestyle just to lose weight. Veganism and vegetarianism aren't diets. They're states of mind, and ways of life. While some people may choose veganism or vegetarianism to lose weight or because they feel it's the "in" thing to do, it's my judgment that such an attitude won't necessarily provide you with the strength of mind to continue on the journey. I'll have more to say about this later. However, what you should know now is that vegetarian women come in many sizes—from women's size 2 to an 18—and men may range from size 28 to 46.

Society today is so stuck on clothing size that we're in danger of missing the entire picture when it comes to food. In my judgment, choosing a vegetarian or vegan lifestyle is all about the quality of our lives and not about the quantity of food we may eat. It's about making healthful eating

DRAMA-FREE MIND AND SPIRIT EXERCISES

1. On a piece of paper, make two columns. Label one vegetarian, the other vegan.
2. Write down why you'd want to become a vegetarian or vegan under the respective columns.
3. Write down next to each reason the pros and cons for *you* becoming a vegetarian or vegan.
4. Reread what you wrote and check off what's important to *you*.
5. You have now made a step of faith to become committed to the lifestyle that lets your individuality shine.
6. Repeat to yourself: *I am a shining star as I step in faith into this* _____ [fill in vegetarian or vegan] *lifestyle.*

choices and exercising daily. Just because you may be a larger vegetarian or vegan doesn't mean you're not healthy. After all, you may be an athlete, and need muscle to bulk up. More to the point, when we focus on the size of our clothing in deciding whether to become a vegetarian, we miss the positive quality of these lifestyles. We should choose vegetarianism because it compliments who we are, what we stand for, and reflects

DRAMA-FREE EXERCISE FOR THE BODY

Stop weighing yourself daily. Weigh yourself once a week instead. The scale is not a true indication of your weight loss. As we exercise, our bodies tone up and the fat turns to muscle, which is heavier but healthier. The scale may say we gained two pounds, but that two pounds may be the muscle we've acquired through regular exercise. Judge your body weight on how your clothes fit, which is a better indication of your size.

our beliefs. Vegetarianism is not a short-term fix or fad, but something that should match our long-term needs and goals.

For whatever reasons we may become vegetarian—an interest in social justice, concern for the welfare of animals, a desire to live lightly on the land, or a wish to have a healthy life—we should take that task seriously *and* enjoy it. We can live with our principles and still have fun in the sun, allow sand to creep between our toes, hike on a cool autumn day, and rollick like a child making angels in the snow. Vegetarianism is all that and more. We need to let our individuality shine through these beautiful lifestyles.

breakfast of champions

VEGAN

I love old-fashioned oatmeal for breakfast. The individual packages of processed, flavored, or microwaved oatmeal don't compare to the oatmeal made on your stovetop. Don't think that you don't have time to make oatmeal for breakfast before you dart off to work. It takes only two to five minutes. That's a short amount of time for a nutritious and satisfying breakfast of champions.

For an alternative oatmeal, I also love the nuttiness and natural texture of steel-cut oats, but any natural oat will do. I like to pick a quality company for my oatmeal. In fact, I like to support smaller food companies that cater to vegetarians. That way, I'm ensured of quality, nongenetically modified ingredients with no extra additives. Small companies that cater to vegetarians tend to make their products with love and care for people and the environment.

Whatever kind of oatmeal you choose to get you through the morning, full and energized, here are my favorite two recipes for breakfast. As I prepare my coffee, I start the water boiling in the pot. As the cereal cooks, I gather my lunch made from the evening before into my lunch bag and get dressed. This way, I don't waste any more time.

Cooking Time: 10 minutes
Serving: 1

Old-Fashioned-Style Oatmeal Ingredients

1 cup of water	2 tbsp organic ground flaxseed
1/2 cup of old-fashioned-style oatmeal	1 tbsp peanuts or any nut variety
	1 tbsp raisins

Old-Fashioned-Style Oatmeal Directions

1. Boil water in a pot.
2. Once water boils, add all the rest of the ingredients. Stir.
3. Turn down heat and simmer for seven to ten minutes, until oatmeal is of desired consistency.
4. Serve in a fun bowl for a cheerful start to your day.

Steel-Cut Oats Ingredients

3/4 cup of water	1 tbsp peanuts or any nut variety
1/4 cup of steel-cut oats	2 tbsp organic ground flaxseed
2 tbsp raisins	

Steel Cut Oats Directions

1. Boil water in a pot.
2. Once water boils, add all the rest of the ingredients. Stir.
3. Turn down heat and simmer for six to seven minutes.
4. Serve in a fun bowl for a cheerful start to your day!

DAY 7

congratulations! one full week completed!

If you grew up in the 1970s, you may remember seeing everywhere a poster that featured a cute, fuzzy kitten clinging onto a tree branch. Under the kitten were the words, "Hang in there." The poster is still around. Even today, you'll see some variation of it—whether in your manager's office, on a nearby desk, or in your college dorm. It's a good message. Hang in there!

You've just completed a full week as a vegetarian! That's an accomplishment to be proud of. Although completing the first day as a vegetarian was an achievement, completion of a full week is a triumph. Whether you completed the first week without falling off the path, or you stumbled and got right back up, you're a success and I'm proud of you. You should be proud of yourself. Say it: *I am a vegetarian and I am proud of myself for completing a full week!* You go with your bad self!

DRAMA-FREE MIND AND SPIRIT EXERCISES

1. Check off completing a full week as a vegetarian from your goal list. It feels good! Give yourself a hug. Wrap your arms around yourself and hug yourself. Loving yourself starts with you first, and no one else. If you can't love yourself, you can't expect someone else to love who you are. Love for yourself means having completed this first full week to take back your health.
2. Write down your next goal, if you haven't already, and use this good feeling today as your fuel to continue your journey.
3. Write down the good feeling you're experiencing right now. Then, when you feel a difficult time coming on in your vegetarian journey, you can reread how you felt on completing a week and how you got to that point. This will keep you focused and strong in walking the vegetarian path.

Keep that positive energy going. It's your fuel to complete another day, another week, a month, two months, six months, a year, two years, and more. Praise yourself. Congratulate yourself. Remember when I spoke on goals for Day 2? Completion of the first week as a vegetarian should have been one of them. Maybe it was your seventh goal if you were setting a goal each day; maybe it was your second, and just completing the first day was your first. Whatever number this goal was, you made it! You were like the little engine that said, "I think I can . . . I think I can." But you went further, and said, "I know I can . . . I know I can!" You did this by yourself with faith, strength, and courage.

Give yourself a hug, a round of applause. Tell yourself that you love yourself for what you did. Such a feeling will carry you through the good and bad times—when those meat cravings are at their strongest. (Read Day 8 on cravings to continue to stay strong.) Being a vegetarian is living as though your body is your temple and your life is your palace.

DRAMA-FREE EXERCISE FOR THE BODY

You're feeling so good right now that you should take that energy and go for a walk, run, bike, start a vegetable/herb garden, or something outdoors that will power up your body, mind, and spirit with even more good feelings. My best workouts are when I'm filled with joy and laughter.

Your life is your "palace" because you are positively caring for your body, mind, and spirit; your body is a temple capable of healing itself, and providing a defense against diseases. Take back your health by living a wonderful full week and more of the vegetarian lifestyle!

DRAMA-FREE EASY RECIPE

celebration black-eyed peas stew

VEGAN

Black-eyed peas are a traditional part of Southern culture, especially among African Americans. On New Year's Day, my mother would cook a pot of black-eyed pea soup for lunch to bring us luck, and add greens for monetary wealth. Apparently, the New Year tradition of eating black-eyed peas for good fortune didn't start in the American South, but was introduced by Jews celebrating Rosh Hashanah, the Jewish New Year.

Whatever its origins, this delicious, nutty-tasting meal transcends all cultures and is a favorite of many. Let's celebrate your first full week as a vegetarian by using this recipe. I've combined both "good luck" traditions of greens and black-eyed peas for a celebratory meal! After all, a celebration of a full week as a vegetarian is similar to a "New Year" for you! May you have good luck and prosperity—and I know you will—on your continued journey!

Cooking Time: 60–65 minutes
Servings: 6–8

Ingredients

8 cups of water

1 16-oz. package of dry black-eyed peas (cleaned, rinsed, soaked per package instructions)

1 large onion, chopped

4 garlic cloves, diced

1 tbsp ground chipotle pepper

2 cups celery, chopped

2 tbsp olive oil

1 tbsp dried Italian seasoning

2 cups frozen okra

Three cans diced, roasted garlic tomatoes (not drained)

1 tsp seasoning salt

1/2 tsp ground pepper

1 10–12 oz. package of frozen mustard greens, turnip greens, or collard greens

Optional: Serve with Sister's Spicy Mexican Cornbread Recipe

Directions

1. Boil water.
2. Add dry black-eyed peas to water.
3. Lower heat to simmer and cook for forty-five minutes.

4. While peas are cooking, in a large pan sauté the onions, garlic, and chipotle pepper on medium heat.

5. Add the remaining ingredients, except the greens and cups of water. Stir and lower heat to a simmer. Cook for ten minutes. Set aside.

6. Add ingredients in pan to pot of peas and water after forty-five minutes. Cook for an additional fifteen minutes or longer, until peas are tender.

7. Add the greens to the pot. Stir. Heat for five minutes or until greens are hot.

8. Serve in pasta/soup-style bowls with a side dish of cornbread.

DAY 8

yes, you will crave meat

I won't lie to you, and say that your cravings for meat will magically vanish when you become a vegetarian. Sister Vegetarian tells the truth, and, as the elderly women of my childhood church would say during Sunday morning sermons, "Shame the devil!" After all, I'm a living representative of that temptation. However, what I'll also do is provide you with the tools that will not only make you a stronger person, but a stronger vegetarian or vegan.

I consider myself a strong person. But at least initially in my vegetarian journey, the smell of meat brought back memories: of BBQs hosted by family and friends; of Thanksgiving and Christmas dinners as a child; of chowing down on a Dagwood sandwich piled high with slices of roast beef, ham, turkey, and cheese in my favorite New Jersey delicatessen, or while watching the Yankees on television. You may find yourself responding to the aroma lingering under your nose when passing a restaurant or want to lick your fingers after observing the ribs at a picnic

DRAMA-FREE MIND AND SPIRIT EXERCISES

1. Write down the positive changes you're experiencing and seeing as a vegetarian—ones that you and others are witnessing.
2. Let those wonderful points be your fuel, to attack the cravings head-on and say *no* to meat.
3. If someone asks you if you crave meat as a vegetarian, be honest. Hold your head high and proud: "Yes, I'm only human; *but,* let me tell you why I say *no.*"

surrounded by meat eaters. Don't get mad at Sister! I'm just telling the truth.

I'm here to tell you, however, that you'll have the strength to resist. Not only do you see changes to your health and bodily appearance as a vegetarian, but your attitude changes. You become at peace with yourself and your choice of diet. When you realize that you're no longer confined to bed or filled with medication from viruses that invaded your body so easily as a meat eater; or that you've reversed your type 2 diabetes and heart disease and are now down to fewer or no medications under a physician's care; or, as in my case, the stomach problems that ailed you for over a decade disappear . . . you'll have the courage, strength, tenacity, vigor, energy, self-belief, and faith to just say *No!* You'll know that by saying *no* to meat you're extending your life and becoming healthier.

In fact, you'll become so filled with energy that you'll be unstoppable. You'll remember that I mentioned that I began running once again after I became a vegetarian; and, eventually running a half marathon. Let me go into more detail. In my late twenties and early thirties I ran solely for exercise and as relief for stress. However, in my twenties, when I ate meat, I could only run up to three miles before I ran out of breath. In my early thirties, when I dabbled in vegetarianism for almost a year, I ran up to eight miles, but then ended up hurting myself from pushing too fast, too soon. I stopped running and returned to hiking and backpacking. When I entered my forties, I decided to try running, but huffed and puffed through one mile, stopping at five miles. I felt like I was having a heart attack.

When I became a vegetarian, I discovered energy. I decided to try running again at age forty-four. I ran three miles and felt good. The next weekend, I ran four. The next week, I ran three miles during the workweek, then five miles on the weekend. In two months, I was up to ten miles on the weekend, and would increase my mileage by running three to six miles before work. In addition to my weekly runs, I rode on my stationary bike once a week for an hour at a pace of twelve m.p.h. I hiked or backpacked on a Saturday and ran a long-distance run over twelve miles on a Sunday.

Once I became a vegetarian, I found myself neither tired nor exhausted after a mile of running, biking, or hiking. I'd only give myself two days of nonconsecutive rest a week, and still I did not tire. Within two-and-a-half months of beginning my running program, I could run twelve or more miles nonstop without being tired. I started to take part in races. I joined a women's beginner runners group. I also trained on my own, running races every other week.

DRAMA-FREE EXERCISE FOR THE BODY

You may crave meat, but a vegetarian lifestyle gives you more energy to perform athletically. Don't worry if you can't walk, run, or bike a mile yet. Stick with the vegetarian path, and you'll be going farther with renewed zest and energy. Set exercise goals for yourself that you can stick with. One goal may be to walk a half mile for a few weeks, and increase it by a half mile every two weeks. When you crave meat, remember you're becoming stronger and are able to exercise longer with a vegetarian lifestyle. You'll have more energy to reach your exercise goal as a vegetarian rather than as a meat eater. The choice is yours. I know you'll decide on more energy to be all you can be!

Finally, a little over a year after completing my first year of drama-free vegetarian living, I ran my first half marathon, completing it in two hours and twenty-one minutes, without stopping and walking once. For someone who'd never run cross-country at school, and for whom the very concept of running 13.1 miles a year before would have been laughable, I exceeded all my expectations. Not only did I feel as though I picked up energy and speed during the course of the race, but I found myself becoming more confident, and positive thoughts were filling my mind. Not only was I doing something I'd thought impossible only twelve months previously, but I was debunking myths that vegetarians don't have enough energy, stamina, or strength to compete.

As I ran, I even waved and jumped up and down with glee at spectators and a camera crew. I hollered for others and myself. I began to pass other men and women en route and cheered them on and offered them encouraging words. Thirty seconds from the finishing line I broke into a sprint, to emphasize to myself that my second chance in life was not going to be taken lightly.

All this is to say that, although you may crave meat initially in your journey, you'll develop the physical and mental resources to resist it. You'll gain energy and strength that will allow you to compete successfully, even when you thought you were too old and/or unfit to do so. The temptations of meat—the smell, and remembered taste and texture—won't go away. Indeed, it's okay to be human and crave it—after all, you may have been eating it most of your life. The point is not to be too hard on yourself, but to think how your life will change, or has changed, as a vegetarian. Acknowledge the temptation, but list the positives.

uncle joe's cuban sandwich

LACTO-OVO VEGETARIAN (WITH VEGAN VERSION)

When I was a kid, for two months of the summer vacation, two weeks of my school's Christmas holiday, and one week of my Easter break, my mother and I would travel from New Jersey to California. We struggled as a family, but my mother wanted to make sure I knew my maternal family. In California, we'd visit with my mother's mother, grandmother, sisters, aunts, and uncles. Sometimes during the summer, Mom would send my sister and me, and come later. She wanted me to know who I was, and I appreciated her for that.

My uncle Joe of Benicia, California, was my all-time favorite uncle. He lived near my grandmother, and I'd jump up and down pleading with her to let me walk five minutes down the road to hang out with Uncle Joe. From the age of five through eleven, I would sit for hours with him in his high-backed chair while Bobby "Blue" Bland, B. B. King, and other great blues singers played on his record player. He had 75s, 45s, and LPs, and it's because of him that I discovered my love of blues and jazz. Uncle Joe would compare one great singer to another, and sing along—responding to the music with "That's right!" or "Oh, yeah . . . say it!"

So much did I love my uncle Joe that my grandmother would have to call his house several times to get me back home. Sometimes she'd threaten my hide, but Uncle Joe always had my back, and promised me that I could return later that day or tomorrow. I call this sandwich Uncle Joe's Cuban Vegetarian Sandwich because it's so cool, soulful, bluesy, jazzy, and just fun—like Uncle Joe. It fulfills those meat cravings by representing the many vegetarian sandwiches that are better than the meat versions. This version is hip without knowing it. Just sitting on your plate, it's cool. It's Uncle Joe's coolness!

Preparation and Cooking Time: 20–30 minutes
Servings: 1

Ingredients

Olive oil

2 inch-thick slices of fresh eggplant (if you prefer, use one large portobello mushroom cap)

Vegan liquid smoke

1 Italian hard roll, sliced open

2 tbsp Cuban Aioli Sauce (recipe below)

2 slices of bread and butter sandwich stuffer pickles

1/2 cup of roasted peppers (I use roasted peppers in a jar)

2 slices of fresh mozzarella cheese (use vegan mozzarella cheese for a vegan version)

1 slice of onion, sliced in rounds and cut in half to break apart

1/2 avocado, chopped

Aioli Sauce Ingredients

1 Hass avocado, halved, pitted, and peeled

1/4 cup vegan mayonnaise

1 tbsp lemon juice

4 medium garlic cloves, peeled

1–2 chipotle peppers halves in adobo sauce, depending on how hot you prefer the sauce

1/2 cup mustard greens leaves

1/2 tsp sea salt

1/2 tsp vegan liquid smoke

Aioli Sauce Directions

Mix all ingredients above in a food processor. Store in an airtight container, or a glass jar. It keeps in the refrigerator for five to seven days.

Uncle Joe's Cuban Sandwich Directions

1. Place oven on broil.
2. Lightly grease pan in olive oil.
3. Place eggplant slices or mushroom on pan. Drizzle with vegan liquid smoke.
4. Broil four minutes on each side.
5. Take out of oven and set aside.
6. Slice open hard rolls, and press down with hand to flatten both sides of roll.
7. Spread each roll with 1 tbsp Aioli sauce on each roll.
8. Add eggplant or mushroom on one side.
9. Add roasted peppers, cheese (regular or vegan), onions, and avocado.
10. Place other roll on top.
11. Lightly oil a small pan with olive oil.
12. Preheat a small pan on medium heat.
13. Add sandwich, and place a small saucer on sandwich top to press sandwich down. A Cuban sandwich is pressed almost flat.
14. Flip sandwich once bottom roll becomes crusty.
15. Place saucer back on other side of roll as other bottom becomes crusty.
16. Remove and serve.

Ooh! So soulful, cool, jazzy, and bluesy!

DAY 9

hey . . . good lookin'

In the 1980s, the all-female group Klymaxx released the song "The Men All Pause," which encouraged me and other women to feel good about ourselves, no matter our size or facial features. As a college freshman, I would place the record on the turntable and dance on my bed in my dorm as my roommate laughed at my craziness.

I loved that song not only for the encouragement it gave women, but for how the women in the band of various sizes could look totally fierce, beautiful, and strong at the same time. Before the 1980s, it was rare to see women who weren't only lead or back-up singers. Klymaxx consisted of six women of color who played their own instruments: drums, bass, lead guitar, and keyboard. And they all could belt out a serious tune! I was shy, but they weren't. I was learning to be strong, and they were strong women with an anthem that I loved singing. These six women said, in effect: "It's okay to be strong and look good. It's okay to celebrate our beauty, and still be individuals. It's okay to be individualists and unique."

Contrary to what myths you may have heard about vegetarians, we too can be sexy or handsome. We can be toned, muscular, and curvy. In fact, as the saying goes, "We're all that and a bag of chips!" Being a vegetarian doesn't mean sitting in the lotus position all day or wearing sackcloth! Get a manicure or pedicure; wear funky shoes and clothing that show off your curvaceous or muscular body; get a chic haircut or "do"; and simply celebrate the sexiness or handsomeness of you. You deserve

DRAMA-FREE MIND AND SPIRIT EXERCISES

1. I purchased my designer shoes and underwear in a sale. If you're budgeting, shop around for inexpensive designer names. The designer names last longer due to quality, but there's no need to spend the original price and go bankrupt. Be a cautious shopper to end up with more in your bag, and more left in your bank account.

2. If you cannot afford weekly manicures or pedicures, do them yourself. I do my own pedicures and experiment with fun, funky colors and easy self-adhesive decals. I use the pack of peel-on pictures for manicures and pedicures that can be bought inexpensively at any beauty supply store. People actually thought I had a professional pedicure because of the designs on my toes.

3. Here's a secret. Do you want a Swedish, sports, or therapeutic massage that costs half the price? Go to a massage school. You'll pay around half the price for a massage that's professionally done by students nearing graduation. Every massage school has a clinic open to the public. The only difference between a professional spa and a school-massage clinic is that you may not have a fireplace to sit at before or after your massage as you're wrapped in a thick, soft spa robe and drink an herbal tea! Yes, it sounds comfortable; but I'm paying for a massage to relax my muscles after running or hiking. I don't care about the extras. Decide on what matters to you; but take care of your temple with a form of relaxation to replenish and reenergize.

DRAMA-FREE EXERCISE FOR THE BODY

Have fun with exercise. Purchase fun and funky workout clothing for running, biking, walking, hiking, or whatever you choose to do as an exercise. Looking good as you exercise is a good motivator, and it forces you to go out and show off that new, cool outfit!

to love your body, and love yourself in your body.

The key to being a successful vegetarian is to love the skin you're in. Be proud of the changes happening inwardly and outwardly. Look good as a vegetarian. Even if I'm wearing cargo pants, as when I'm hiking and backpacking, I'm "lookin' good" because I'm celebrating who I am. I recently purchased designer shoes with four-and-a-half-inch heels, and sexy underwear to show off my sexiness to myself and then to my husband. When what you wear under your clothes is sexy, your confidence shines through to the surface and permeates all aspects of your life. Others see that confidence in you. To love ourselves, we need to love the body we're in. This means loving our bodies at every weight. As vegetarians we're healthy and strong. We are fierce. We are strong. We are unique. Each of us is an individual worthy of loving ourselves and being loved. Show off that sexy vegetarian body, no matter your size. Be proud of it, and look good doing it!

spicy mexican cornbread

VEGAN

Do you know what's "lookin' good" all dressed up? Sister's Spicy Mexican Cornbread. This is not your typical cornbread: it's spicy, sensual, sexy, and of course delicious. Eat this with Sister's Celebration Black-eyed Pea Stew (Day 7) or the Vegetarian Chili (Day 13).

Preparation and Mixing Time: 5–7 minutes
Baking Time: 30–35 minutes
Serving Size: 12–15 individual cornbreads

Ingredients

2 cups cornmeal

1 cup wheat flour

1/2 tsp baking soda

1/2 tsp cornstarch

1/3 cup vegetable oil

1/4 cup maple syrup

1 cup vegan sour cream

1 cup of rice milk (alternatives: hemp milk, coconut milk, or soymilk)

2 tsp raw apple cider vinegar

1 cup of frozen corn, defrosted

1 finely chopped medium chili pepper (leave vein and seeds, unless you prefer less spicy)

1/2 tsp vegan liquid smoke

Directions

1. Preheat oven to 350 degrees F.
2. Grease a 9-inch x 13-inch glass baking pan.
3. In a bowl, mix all dry ingredients.
4. Make a well in center of bowl and add wet ingredients.
5. Mix all ingredients well.
6. Place in baking pan.
7. Bake forty to forty-five minutes, until a toothpick comes out clean.
8. Cool down enough to slice without crumbling. Slice into squares. Serve warm.

Tip: I store leftover cornbread in freezer bags and place them in my freezer. Reheat individual servings in an oven or microwave.

DAY 10

yes, you can still have a fly and phat ass

Any physical exercise combined with a healthful vegetarian lifestyle supports and maintains optimum health physically, mentally, and spiritually. In addition, you'll have and be able to maintain an awesome "phat," fit, and beautiful body. *Phat* is a slang word that's used to describe anything attractive or appealing. When the word's applied to a person's physique, it usually means that a woman has a beautifully curvaceous body with "plenty of hips and thighs." If you're a phat guy, you have a body that makes the person giving the comments want to melt in your arms!

Sad to say, many women hear comments from family, friends, spouses, boyfriends, and others that say, in effect, "If you become a vegetarian, you'll lose your phat ass . . . " or, "Don't exercise, you'll lose your ass." Men also hear that they'll lose their muscle tone. Like all myths, these

DRAMA-FREE MIND AND SPIRIT EXERCISES

1. Purchase a pair of jeans or an outfit that you want to wear at your goal weight, if you're planning to lose weight. Use this outfit as your goal, and it's your reward. As your inches melt away weekly, you'll gradually see your progress, as you begin to fit into your new outfit.

2. Reward yourself monthly with new lingerie—something so sexy that only you know you're wearing it at work, school, or anywhere around town. It's for your eyes only, and no one else but you. You'll feel so good and sexy that you'll want to stick to your vegetarian lifestyle and exercise program.

3. Loving yourself first is the key to maintaining a vegetarian lifestyle and exercise program.

observations aren't true. They're simply comments aimed by those who don't want you to succeed! They want you to maintain the status quo of living unhealthily, and bring you down with them. Misery loves company. That's too much drama for me.

The good news is that you can resist this drama, by knowing that the notion that you'll fade to nothingness is and will always be a myth. So, let's move on to the good news of keeping that phat body.

As I noted on Day 9, when you become a vegetarian, you can still maintain your curvaceous or muscular body—except your phat ass and muscles are now toned and firm. All eyes are on you and mouths drop in envy as you cross the room in your new vegetarian and exercised-fit body at family and friend gatherings.

Of course, some people may be trying to make you feel good, such as when they say, "I love you the way you are. So why change?" All you have to do is acknowledge their concern and continue with your plan. It's funny how those comments change when they see your new, physically fit body:

"Damn!" You look good!"

"Baby, I knew you had to tone up, but I just wanted it to be your idea."

"Baby, do you want to celebrate that body?"

"I bought you a little something . . . from Victoria's Secret."

"You know baby, your body would look good in those _____."

"Girl, your bottom is to die for!"

Oh yes, the comments can go on! Of course, that individual may take credit for your transformation, as if they supported you all the way or even came up with the idea. But you'll have to overlook their nerve, smile right back at them, and enjoy the comments—as hard as it might be not to remind them that they were against your changing. Gloat, if you want. You made it through the drama and negative comments on your body and came out looking good!

My drama-free advice is to start your vegetarian and exercise program knowing that there are always people who'll have negative comments both before and during your

DRAMA-FREE EXERCISE FOR THE BODY

Start a basic fitness program, if you're not already on an exercise plan. You don't need to join a gym to stay in shape. Save your money, and use what you have already. Walk, run, or bike. Many communities also have softball and basketball leagues for women in their thirties to their sixties and beyond. No experience is usually necessary, and you can stay fit while meeting new people. What's your exercise passion? Are you a closet runner, softball player, marathoner, walker, hiker, backpacker, or biker waiting to come out? Go it alone or join a walking group, running group, hiking group, or other group for fun. It's cheaper than a gym membership, which isn't usually used. Check out meetup.com or your local community center for beginner, intermediate, and advanced exercise programs.

transformation. They may or may not see the before, during, and after phases, but you most definitely will. Picture yourself healthy, toned, and fit, looking phat and fly in your new body—and believe it. Know that you're already there simply by starting a vegetarian lifestyle, and add the exercise program for optimal health benefits.

Don't worry about how long or far you can walk, run, bike, or exercise in general. It's not about "how long" or "how far." It's getting started and continuing the program that counts. It's not about how many times you fail and give up; it's how many times you start it again and maintain it daily, every other day, or weekly that counts. That's the mountain to climb—consistency and tenacity. Take it from me: The view from the top is beautiful.

DRAMA-FREE EASY RECIPE

fly and phat collard greens hummus wrap

VEGAN

Hummus, a dish that originated in Egypt and dates back several thousand years, is a spread that's ubiquitous in cuisine from the Middle East and North Africa. For lacto-ovo vegetarians to hard-core vegans, hummus is the queen of quick meals, snacks, and appetizers. Hummus is made from chickpeas (aka garbanzo beans) and is stylish all by itself; but when she's dressed up with collard greens she makes a regal, phat entrance!

When you find that tortillas, pita, or chapatis have become too monotonous, collard greens are perfect for a fat-free sandwich wrap. Collard green leaves are sturdy and wide enough to hold their own as a substitute for flour-based sandwich holders. They're also an excellent source of antioxidants, calcium, and vitamins that protect against deformities and cancer.

Hummus is an incredibly versatile dish, and you can basically make the recipe your own by adding ingredients such as roasted bell peppers, chipotle pepper, more or less garlic, more or less tahini, natural peanut butter instead of tahini, spinach, artichokes, sundried tomatoes, beets, turnip roots, and so on. You can also blend hummus to make it as smooth, creamy, or chunky as you like. I prefer my hummus somewhere between smooth and chunky.

Preparation Time: 20 minutes
Servings: 5

Ingredients

1 15-oz. can chickpeas, drained

1 tbsp dried parsley or 2 tbsp fresh parsley

3 tbsp chopped onions

1 tbsp Bragg's Liquid Aminos (*Note*: excellent source of non-genetically modified protein)

1/4 cup tahini (besides whole foods type stores, many grocery stores now put tahini in the health food section. But if tahini is still hard to find, use natural organic peanut butter in its place.)

3 cloves of garlic

1/3 cup of lemon juice

1 1/2 tsp ground cumin (*optional*: instead of cumin, try ground curry, as it adds an even stronger spiciness)

1/4 tsp ground chipotle pepper (*optional*: adds a nice smoky pepper flavor)

2 to 3 drops of vegan liquid smoke for additional smokiness

Set Aside to Stuff Sandwich
Collard greens leaves for the wrap

Directions

Mixing Hummus

Process all the above ingredients (except the collard green leaves and sandwich stuffers) in a food processor or blender until smooth or the consistency you prefer.

Wrapping Hummus

Start with the wrap. After cleaning the collard, cut off the large end of the stem. I slice down the leaf in the center of the large vein. Sometimes I just keep the leaf whole and wrap the hummus the long way. Whatever you prefer, it's all delicious! Spread hummus on the collard leaves.

Stuffers

You can make your hummus sandwich different every day, depending on your stuffers. Before I roll the collard leaf wrap (or whatever wrap I choose), I stuff my sandwich with spinach or kale leaves, sliced cucumbers, and occasionally raisins and/or nuts. Just be creative, and enjoy the process of putting your love into this quickly made meal! Roll and serve.

DAY 11

courage

The moment you decided to become a vegetarian or vegan required courage: to go against the norm in society, to start by yourself to improve your health, to do it on your own.

Courage was already inside you. You simply brought it to the surface and showed everyone that you have the courage to walk this vegetarian journey in spite of those who'd stop you. Think about other things you've started when all else was against you. You may not have finished them, but you had the courage to start. That deserves applause, because people may *think* about instituting a change in their lives or starting something new but never get in motion. You did.

I myself have started many different projects, but have stopped as soon as I started. One of the biggest reasons I gave up was because I was scared to continue, not knowing what lay ahead of me. I lost faith in myself to achieve. I was so afraid of failing that I'd talk myself out of starting, of even trying. I thought that I didn't have the strength or cour-

DRAMA-FREE MIND AND SPIRIT EXERCISES

1. Think about what you've started and stopped in the past. Write down the reasons why you stopped. Now think about the situation that surrounded you when started. Reflect. You'll realize that you then had courage to start.
2. Fuel yourself with thoughts of the courage that you found out you actually had from the exercise above. Surround yourself with these thoughts and use them as your daily motivator.
3. Place these statements where you can see them—on your refrigerator, bathroom mirror, dresser mirror, workplace, or anywhere. For example, maybe your courage was starting a college program as a single parent or with little funds. You may not have finished yet, but you had the courage to start. Maybe you faced adversity to start something. Read them and let them fuel you. You can! You will!

age. You may have your own examples: of wanting to return to college for a career change after already acquiring a bachelor's degree twenty years prior; you'd like to start a novel but think you'll never finish it; you dream of opening a business but fold when the going gets slightly rough.

What I didn't realize was that I already possessed the strength and courage I needed to succeed just by starting to walk in the direction of those goals. I thought that courage came by sticking it out and finishing what I started. But the courage was there all along. I just needed to know and believe that I already possessed what I needed to succeed.

It was my exercise program that I discussed earlier that showed me I already possessed this courage. I wanted to prove to myself that forty-four was still young, and that I could be as athletic as when I was twenty-something. I wanted to show that being in your forties—or fifties, sixties, seventies, or eighties—is beautiful.

Running also taught me that it wasn't the completion of the journey that motivated me, but the courage to continue through all the drama. Becoming a vegetarian enabled me to discover wonderful things about who I was. It offered me new beginnings, and the exhilaration of this lifestyle rolled into a flood of daily joy, inspiration, and motivation.

Vegetarianism enabled me to recognize that I was the captain of my own ship. I saw that I didn't need anyone else to motivate me and keep me on track. Of course, it would be nice if a friend or family member made up their mind to join you as a companion, sharing advice, recipes, and stories. All these are wonderful to experience. However, as I discovered, they aren't absolutely necessary. As a saying goes, "You are your own best motivator." Indeed, even with your companionship, a friend will need to walk their journey alone.

I should note that vegetarianism is not a race. It's an experience and state of mind that requires attention to notice every astonishing vista. If you think you can sprint to see if you can be the better vegetarian or ultimate vegan, you'll miss out on discovering the inner purpose of the journey, which is to find out who you really are.

You go, my vegetarian sister and brother! Keep on stepping! Keep on believing! Keep on walking in courage!

DRAMA-FREE EXERCISE FOR THE BODY

Rev up your exercise program by adding an enjoyable twist to the mundane: compete in fun races. Do you want to compete walking, running, or biking? It takes courage to compete against others who may or may not be better than you. However, you're actually competing against no one but yourself. Prove to yourself that you have the courage, strength, endurance, and power to do whatever you set your mind to. Running, biking, walking—all have fun races and a chance to meet new friends.

courageous spicy-smoky beet hummus

VEGAN

Be unique and courageous. When you step off the path of society's norms, you discover that you can do many amazing things in your life. That's what this dish is all about: creativity, walking your own path, being courageous. I discovered this recipe by being myself—I love to be creative in the kitchen.

Preparation Time: 25 minutes
Servings: 5

Ingredients

1 15-oz. can chickpeas, rinsed and drained

1 cup of fresh mustard greens chopped rough (leaves mostly left whole)

1/2 raw beet root (cut into one-inch thickness, washed with skin left on for more nutrients)

1/2 medium apple (cut into one-inch thickness, leave skin on)

1/4 tsp smoked paprika

1/2 tsp ground chipotle

1/2 small onion cut in half

3 large whole garlic cloves

1 tbsp Bragg's Liquid Aminos (Note: excellent source of non-genetically modified protein)

1/4 cup organic peanut butter
(Note: hummus traditionally
uses tahini, but I did a twist
and used the popular peanut
butter substitute, which is
less expensive)

1/3 cup lemon juice

1 1/2 tsp ground cumin

1/4 tsp vegan liquid smoke

Directions

Place all the ingredients in a food processor or blender, adding the liquid ingredients first, until smooth or the consistency you prefer.

Serve accordingly to your preference.

Set aside to stuff sandwich: collard green leaves, tortillas, chapati, or flatbread.

Wrap Stuffers Ideas

Diced beets, kale, spinach, cucumbers, sundried tomatoes, raisins, peanuts, or your spark of creativity.

Wrapping Hummus

Starting with the wrap, spread hummus on the wrap. Stuff with desired ingredients. Roll and serve.

DAY 12

don't mess
with my mind

What epitomizes our struggle to become and stay a vegetarian for life, when those around us aren't vegetarians and/or don't support our choices? I've thought a lot about this question. I've slept on it and pondered it, and then it conceptualized itself before my eyes as I was reading through some of the passages I'd highlighted in one of my favorite books, *Standing Tall*. The book, which was written by C. Vivian Stringer, Rutgers University's Scarlet Knights women's basketball coach, details Ms. Stringer's struggles to break down the many barriers to a woman of color and how she became one of the top female women's basketball coaches in the world. It was a book that touched me deeply, and it might as well be titled "Keys to Success in Life in All that You Do." One of the theories that Ms. Stringer elaborated was that of the "strong mind."

In 1972, Ms. Stringer was the coach of Cheyney University's basketball team. Cheyney was a small, historically black college in Pennsylvania whose teams were going up against colleges and universities with much larger sports budgets. Coach Stringer told her team that they may not have the resources of the bigger colleges, but that they were strong in their minds, and that no one could influence them because they knew who they were.

This is my message to you.

Possessing a strong mind can prevent anyone from changing your mind about your vegetarian journey. When your mind is strong, a gust of wind cannot blow you down and turn your world upside down. In fact, a gale is ineffective. Neither a whisper in your ear, nor a conversation you overhear, nor your friend saying "Just have a small taste, baby . . . it won't hurt you . . . you can eat healthy tomorrow," will shift you, knock you down, turn your head, or place that meat in your mouth. When we're strong, no one can stop us if we know what we want, where we're going, and what is best for us. Strong minds have shaped history. They shape the present and future. Shape your vegetarian present and future with a healthy, strong mind.

I've been a vegetarian before—in 1996. I was gung-ho serious. I was

DRAMA-FREE MIND AND SPIRIT EXERCISES

1. Reinforce a strong mind by repeating to yourself, *Do they know who I am? I am strong and can do all things!* Repeat this. Say it louder. Say it with a smile.

2. Write down positive comeback phrases for various situations that you encounter. If someone makes a comment questioning the health benefits of vegetarianism, or poses the ubiquitous question, "How do you get enough protein?" think of a response. You don't want to increase the negativity. A positive comeback can mean you change someone's life by starting them thinking about becoming a vegetarian.

married at the time to my first husband. I'd make a vegetarian dish for myself, then cook his meals of meat. Although my husband didn't say, "Have a bite of this steak," he'd nonetheless exclaim, "Mmm! This steak is great! Too bad you're a vegetarian. . . . You don't know what you're missing. But keep eating, baby . . . it's just not for me. . . . " After a year, I gave up vegetarianism. I cooked a sixteen-ounce T-bone steak drizzled with a garlic and butter sauce. At the time, I thought I was in heaven. Now, as I look back on that moment, I regret not standing firm. However, if I hadn't had that experience, I wouldn't have been able to relate to your struggle to become and keep being a vegetarian, when family, friends, and coworkers aren't helping.

Before I realized that you must believe in yourself, that small breath in my ear would knock me down. My mind was not strong. I couldn't see how people could remain vegetarians and not falter when loved ones weren't. I wanted to save animals, I wanted to be healthy, and I wanted to be a vegetarian, but I couldn't see how I could wall myself off from meat eaters and society at large.

After 1996, I continued to waver for years. My current husband and soul mate is supportive—now; he wasn't so initially, because I was weak. Once I became stronger and confident in my vegetarian journey, he respected who I was as a vegetarian. He wanted me to succeed because he saw the belief and confidence I had in myself. People love to observe other people, and they can see if you're weak or strong. We give off positive and negative, as well as strong and weak, vibes through our actions and speech. People will treat you as you project.

Now I can maintain a vegetarian lifestyle knowing that, no matter what people say, I am strong in my mind. I live the evidence of the health benefits of vegetarianism and my own personal experience. I've read the information about how cruelly farmed animals are treated, and how their flesh is injected with hormones and antibiotics to make them grow fast. These facts help strengthen my purpose. Mainly, however, I live by example and practice what I speak. We're all role models because people watch what we do; so let's be positive and healthy ones.

DRAMA-FREE EASY RECIPE

don't mess with my pesto!

VEGAN

Pesto is an Italian, fresh herb-garlic-cheese sauce traditionally served with pasta. I substitute nutritional yeast for Parmesan to make this meal vegan. Nutritional yeast is also an excellent source of protein and B-complex vitamins. It has a nutty and cheesy flavor.

As you know, Sister loves her greens. I don't prepare greens in the traditional U.S. Southern method. I take world and local recipes, and use the greens of my Southern and African-American heritage—the mustard greens, turnip greens, beets, Swiss chard, and collards—to replace basil, parsley, cilantro, and other herbs. In this recipe, I took the beautiful and wonderful Italian pesto and made it with mustard greens.

Mustard greens have a natural peppery taste. See for yourself how delicious they taste by taking a bite of a raw mustard leaf! I love raw mustard greens as a salad; in place of regular lettuce they make a nice accompaniment to this pasta meal. The best part of mustard greens is that they naturally promote heart and lung health, and the uses of this pesto are endless. Try turnip greens in place of the mustard greens; or make it with half mustard and half turnip greens! Borrow from Southern and African-American culinary heritage for a nutritional and delicious twist to your meals.

Preparation Time: 10–15 minutes
Servings: Makes 1 cup

Ingredients

3 cups of raw mustard greens (leaves and stems on, do not chop)

1/4 cup extra virgin olive oil, or more if pesto is too dry after blending

5–6 medium-size garlic cloves (I am a garlic freak, so the more garlic the merrier for me)

1/4 tsp sea salt

1/4 cup peanuts (I always have peanuts on hand, but traditionally pine nuts or walnuts are used)

1/2 cup of nutritional yeast

Directions

1. Process all ingredients in a food processor until well blended, not smooth.
2. Place in a bowl and serve as is, or slightly warmed on top of wheat pasta of your choice. The nuttiness of wheat pasta and nutritional yeast, and the peppery flavor of mustard greens pesto, bring a delicious earthiness to your tables.
3. Store pesto in the refrigerator for up to seven days in a tightly covered container. Place olive oil on top of the pesto when storing in order to prevent drying out.

DAY 13

unique and proud

As a vegetarian, you'll be subject to what I call "why myths." (We came across some of them on Day 5.) I call them this not only because they're questions directed at you that begin with *why*—"Why did you choose this lifestyle?" "Why are you giving up meat?" "Why do you want to alienate yourself?"—but because you may be tempted by your own internal questions—"Why *did* I make this decision?" "Why should I be seen as 'different,' 'unique,' 'weird,' or 'crazy'?"

For me, "why myths" are just another form of drama—a way of generating anxiety and negativity. They're myths because they're not based on reality. Vegetarianism is neither unnatural nor unhealthy. It isn't a recent fad, but has been practiced for millennia. Some have argued that our digestive systems are designed mainly to eat a plant-based diet; others have pointed out that we lack the sharp teeth or claws associated with carnivorous animals. Many worthy individuals throughout history have recognized the ethical dimension of not eating animals. But whatever our motivations, as vegetarians we should embrace the proud legacy of thinking seriously about food, and ignore the lies and myths told about this lifestyle.

Another myth about vegetarians is that we're all the same: that we're all vegetarians for the same reason, that we all like the same food, and that we're social misfits and/or walking clichés of weird lifestyles. I like to use an analogy to represent the uniqueness of every individual. Just as many knitted patterns make up a quilt, each unique and each contributing to the overall beauty of the whole, so we make the world beautiful through our unique qualities and our raising awareness that vegetarianism can save our lives and the environment. As vegetarians, we provide talent and ideas to change the world for the better; as vegetarians we embody an alternative and respectful way of relating to our bodies, our planet, and other animals that critiques the thoughtlessness that characterizes so much of the way we eat, use resources, and treat others. We cut

DRAMA-FREE MIND AND SPIRIT EXERCISES

1. Write down what makes you unique and different from others.
2. Write down how you can use that uniqueness and difference to be the best vegetarian you can be.
3. Become an activist. Being unique and different also means that we have a lot to contribute to society to make it better. We all do. Maybe there's something that needs to be changed in your community (remember the grocery store?). Take a stand, and use your qualities and talents to improve the neighborhood.
4. If someone calls you "different," "unique," "weird," or "out there," thank them joyfully for the compliment and show them how you can help them lead a healthier lifestyle. Use the opportunity to uplift others rather than beat them down, as they're trying to do to you. A little encouragement to our fellow human beings goes much further than trying to put each other down.

DRAMA-FREE EXERCISE FOR THE BODY

Knitting and crocheting constitute exercise, too—a workout for your mind and soul. The purpose of these age-old crafts is to relax and rejuvenate, as well as produce beautiful and useful items. I taught myself to knit through books and videos on the web at the age of forty. I then taught others at work. In a year, I was knitting sweaters, socks, and lacey shawls.

through the myths and labels that determine how we should act and what we should be.

Our uniqueness and difference can inspire others, especially young people, to be authentically who they are, and to bring their own special skills and personality to the great quilt of our society. We can use our positive influence to encourage difference, rather than turn us into bland automata, all following received wisdom and possessing as much personality and insight as a Stepford wife.

I don't know about you, but I don't want to merge into the crowd. I am as real as real can get. I am proud to be different and to contribute ideas that can change my community. If that means being called "unique," "different," "crazy," "weird," or "out there," then I wear those adjectives with honor and just keep moving toward my goal. I am what I am: A proud vegetarian. Are you? Or are you someone who only wants to conform to what society thinks you should be or eat?

great-grandma's proud virginia diner chunky vegetarian chili

VEGAN (WITH LACTO-VEGETARIAN OPTION)

As I mentioned in the Day 2 recipe ("Just Like Grandma Vegan Cinnamon-Raisin Wheat Bread"), my great-grandmother, Otis Mae Robinson, owned a diner in Vallejo, California, in the 1940s and 1950s. My mother told me that the diner's signature dish was a chili, which my mother also prepared to keep her family warm and full of nutrients during the cold New Jersey winters. I dedicate this recipe to Otis Mae, who proudly gave her signature love to her chili recipe at The Virginia Diner. I've changed the recipe to be vegetarian; but the ingredients are similar. This chili was served with love and pride to my family, and now you can do the same to yours.

Cooking Time: 32 minutes
Servings: 4–5

Ingredients

2 tbsp olive oil

1 cup onions, chopped

4 cloves garlic, minced

1 cup of green peppers, chopped

2 15 1/2-oz. cans black beans, drained and rinsed

1 16-oz. package of tofu, drained, and chopped in half-inch to one-inch cubes

1 cup frozen corn

2 slices chipotle peppers in adobo sauce, diced

2 tbsp cacao powder

2 15 1/2-oz. cans of diced roasted tomatoes (do not drain)

2 tbsp raw apple cider vinegar

1 tbsp smoked paprika

1 tbsp ground chipotle pepper

1 cup mustard greens, chopped

Vegan sour cream (use plain organic yogurt if you prefer the lacto-vegetarian option)

Directions

1. Add the olive oil to a large pot. Sauté onions, garlic, green peppers for two minutes.
2. Add the remaining ingredients, except the mustard greens, and bring to a boil.
3. Simmer and cook for twenty-five minutes.
4. Add the greens, and cook for five more minutes.
5. Serve in individual pasta/soup dishes.
6. Serving suggestions: Add a side dish of Spicy Mexican Cornbread. Add a dollop of vegan sour cream or organic plain yogurt on top of each serving of chili if desired.

DAY 14

keep it simple

Earlier, I talked about taking small steps on your path to vegetarianism. Now I'd like to add: Keep it simple. Being a vegetarian doesn't need to be hard. Keep it simple and you'll succeed at your own pace. When we try to imitate others rather than follow our own path, we complicate things needlessly and make it harder for us to focus on what will help *us* to succeed as vegetarians and meet our own needs. After all, we may not yet be ready to take the next step or be reaching toward their goals. Why focus on being an ethical vegan who only eats organic food or a raw foodist, if you know that you're not ready and will simply find it too hard? Make your own path. It's okay to borrow ideas and recipes, and ask others what did or didn't work for them, but you should make this journey your own.

That's how to keep it simple. I speak from experience when I say that many vegetarians fail within the first weeks or months on our path because we try to complicate things too soon or we're walking a path we don't really want to be on at that point in our lives. I've failed many

DRAMA-FREE MIND AND SPIRIT EXERCISES

1. Have fun in creating varied meals. Take all the time you need. You already are a vegetarian. You've been successful just by starting this journey. You just want to see what path you'd like to follow.
2. It's okay to switch back and forth between the varied types of vegetarianism and veganism. You don't live in a dictatorship. No one's going to lock you up if you change. Those who attempt to slap you down need to question who they are; you don't. You are a successful vegetarian, so have some fun.
3. Have a vegetarian and vegan party. Invite friends over to sample meals from different countries, or recipes you created. Use the recipes in this book.
4. Being a vegetarian and vegan is all about fun. If it's not fun, then you're complicating things. Keep it simple and joyful. Keep smiling through it all. It's all about the journey, not the end.

times in the past because I wanted to *start* as a vegan, and I wasn't ready (cheese was my kryptonite). I thought veganism was what I *should* be, and that my vegetarian lifestyle wouldn't make a difference unless I was a vegan. But I wasn't ready.

We need to be who we are. Whether you're a vegetarian who eats dairy products, or someone who eats eggs, or both; whether you're a strict vegetarian or vegan, or a raw foodist—whatever you are, make sure that you're on the path that's right for you. Your admiration for another vegetarian or vegan may have started you on the path to changing your lifestyle, and it's okay to explore the many sides of vegetarianism. But no one should force you into something that doesn't fit your goals or lifestyle. This is *your* journey, and whatever path you choose within vegetarianism or veganism, it should be your choice and decision and no one else's. You should ignore anyone—whether vegan or omnivore—who tells you that your vegetarian or vegan lifestyle is wrong.

I say this simply because you'll be much more likely to stay on the path toward your goals if you're fully confident and invested in the choices you make. When you make it simple, you have peace of mind. Peace of mind creates an environment of success and creativity within our journey. In my case, I finally felt I was ready to be a vegan after a year of being a vegetarian, and after I discovered that cheese was not my kryptonite! It was a choice that suited *my* needs and not someone else's decision. Keep it *simple*, and keep it *real*!

DRAMA-FREE EASY RECIPE

simple after-work sautéed beets and garlic served over pasta and greens

VEGAN

I like to keep my workday meals simple and quick. Although I enjoy preparing meals, after a long day at work I prefer to make a dinner that enables me to have a full evening for myself with my husband. Vegetables and pasta to the rescue! Don't be afraid of the carbohydrates in pasta. Our bodies need good carbs to replenish the energy expended during the day, and to refuel us for the next. If you're an active person who participates in a daily exercise program, then complex carbs from a source such as whole-wheat pasta are your best bet to reenergize tired muscles. I've found that, after some training days for upcoming races, I need solid fuel to replenish my body, give me energy, and keep my digestion working. This quick recipe keeps me full, fit, and fierce!

Cooking Time: Approximately 15 minutes
Servings: 2 (Note: you can expand this meal to three, four, or more servings by adding more pasta and vegetables.)

Ingredients

Two-person serving of wheat spaghetti (I use a spaghetti serving-size measuring tool.)

2 organic beet roots sliced in one-inch pieces, to look like homemade fries (clean beet, but leave the skin on for extra nutrients)

Extra virgin olive oil

4 medium garlic cloves, diced

2 cups fresh turnip greens or beet greens, chopped roughly

Garlic salt and black pepper to taste

(Alternative: instead of beet roots, use turnip roots. Turnip roots have detox properties, and are good for cardiovascular and colon health.)

Directions

1. Boil water for spaghetti. When water is ready, add spaghetti and cook eight to ten minutes until almost al dente, but not yet ready.
2. As pasta cooks, time the sautéing of the sliced beet roots with the cooking of the spaghetti. Heat 2 tbsp of extra virgin olive oil in a saucepan.
3. Add garlic and sliced beet roots to saucepan. Sauté for ten minutes. Season with garlic salt and black pepper to taste.
4. Add the turnip greens or beet greens to the spaghetti and water, and cook for an additional two to four minutes. The pasta should now be al dente and ready to serve, and the turnip greens should be slightly cooked with almost a crunchy texture (as though raw).
5. Drain the pasta and greens. Mix pasta and greens for equal servings before plating.
6. Plate the pasta and greens. Sprinkle a little extra olive oil on spaghetti if desired.
7. Top pasta and greens with the sautéed beets.
8. Serve with heated, sliced, crusty Italian Tuscan bread, drizzled with olive oil if desired.

DAY 15

your family may not always be supportive, but that's okay

I've already mentioned that you may be getting grief from friends and your spouse, parents, grandparents, siblings, cousins, grandchildren, nieces, nephews, aunts, uncles—did I cover everyone? But I think it's worth stating once again that you may get little or no support from the very people whom you thought you could count on through thick and thin. It may be difficult to face this truth, but it's the reality. In this chapter, however, I'm going to dig down a little to uncover the positives in this situation.

You should know that your family still loves you—and that, in fact,

DRAMA-FREE MIND AND SPIRIT EXERCISES

I've found that the best exercise for dealing with family drama is meditation. Sit in a quiet room, or anywhere. (I knew a mother of a five-year-old boy whose only peaceful time away from her son and husband was to sit and meditate in the bathroom for five minutes every morning before work.) I like to burn incense, listen to soft "soundscapes"-type music, such as streams of water, rain falling, or the ocean. (Many cable/digital satellite companies have free music as part of their subscription. "Soundscapes" may include soft violin, guitar, and/or piano-based music, with other peaceful instruments intertwined.)

Breathe deeply and slowly for at least five minutes. Set a timer or your alarm clock for five, ten, fifteen, or more minutes to prevent you from opening and closing your eyes to see how much time has passed. Listen to your breath, and concentrate on your inhalation and exhalation. You'll forget where you are, and enter a trancelike, peaceful state. Once the alarm goes off, take a couple more deep breaths and rise slowly. Your stress will have melted away. You are calm and at peace. No negative comments will touch you.

they *do* have your back when times are tough and you need a lot of loving and praying to get you through the rough spots. But you need to face the fact that your family may not understand why you became a vegetarian, and they're worried that you may have lost your mind. Being family, they're likely to tell you that to your face!

So, what do you do when the following words fly across the room directly at you, and you find yourself looking at your family, just as they're looking at you, as though aliens have taken over their bodies?

DRAMA-FREE EXERCISE FOR THE BODY

By now, you'll know the benefits of an exercise routine in burning excess fat and maintaining a healthy weight. But exercise is also great at reducing stress. A relaxing walk or run during lunchtime or after a hectic day at work can be an excellent stress reducer. Even if you're a morning person like me, and you've already exercised, a quick stroll will calm you down before you say the wrong thing to your workmate, customer, manager, spouse, significant other, friend, or child. De-stress through exercise and your blood pressure will thank you. Your bank balance will thank you, too, because after you went for a walk you decided not to shout at your fellow employee or manager, so you still have a job!

"What! Growing up eating meat is not good enough for you any-
    more?"
"Do you think you're better than us?"
"Meat made you who you are today: healthy! Look, you got a man/
    woman because you ate good growing up!"
"No man/woman wants a skinny woman/man!"
"We did what we could to get by to feed you."
"You will starve!"
"You will lose your butt/muscles."
"Do you want women/men (wife/husband) to stop looking at you?"
"You're going to get too skinny."

And so it goes on . . . and on . . . and on (yawn, yawn). And here's your first defense. I get bored hearing these statements, and so should you. Remember: this is about *your* journey and *your* success. You're not undertaking it to impress your family, to become someone's "favorite" relative, or to keep your position in the family. You don't love your family because of what they eat, and you shouldn't judge their love of you by what you eat. All they're doing is trotting out the myths they've heard from society. They're fearful of change and the unknown, and of their assumptions being challenged. You're bringing an awakening into their lives.

Once family members see how healthy you are, and how many positive physical, spiritual, and mental changes you've brought to your life because of your journey, many may change their views. They may switch to vegetarianism, and start incorporating more vegetarian meals into their diet. Whether they do so, however, or continue to ridicule you is not your concern. You should walk your path with your head held high and not let their comments affect you. Use positive affirmations that announce you still have *victory* on a daily basis. Remember the old adage—"Sticks and stones may break my bones, but words will never hurt me"? It's never been truer than now.

DRAMA-FREE EASY RECIPE

la familia cuban black bean soup

VEGAN

Whether your family supports your vegetarian journey or not, they've still got your back. What better way to celebrate the close-knit families and communities in many Cuban, Puerto Rican, Mexican, Dominican, Haitian, Caribbean, and Louisianan neighborhoods than with a dish common to all of them: black bean soup. Black beans are the heart and soul of many beautiful vegetarian meals from Mexico to Spain, and you can travel the world and experience these many cultures without leaving your kitchen. Each region has their own version of this nutritious, warm, and hearty meal that takes its place on family tables for everyday or celebratory meals.

Black bean soup is very quick and easy to make. Many people are afraid of using dry beans because they think the process is too long. On the contrary, black bean soup really cooks on its own, once the ingredients are added. All you need to do is sit and wait for a beautiful meal that brings families together for laughter, great conversation, and good times.

Cooking Time: 1 hour
Servings: 5–6

Ingredients

1-lb. bag dry black beans (also called turtle beans). Prepare beans overnight, as indicated below.

6 cups of water

4 tbsp extra virgin olive oil

8 garlic cloves, minced

1 onion, chopped fine

1 tsp ground cumin

1 tsp ground curry

1 tsp ground turmeric

1 cup mustard greens, chopped fine

1 tsp smoked paprika

1 tsp ground chipotle pepper

1 cup of frozen, small, cut carrots

1 cup frozen corn

1 cup bell pepper, chopped

1 cup of celery, chopped

1 14 1/2-oz. can diced fire-roasted tomatoes

1 tsp dry Italian seasonings

1/2 tsp sea salt

Brown rice—amount to cook determined by number of servings desired (check package directions)

Directions

Prep Beans Overnight

Rinse beans and soak overnight for at least six hours. If you forgot to soak, or don't have time for the long soaking, boil the beans in water for one to three minutes, turn off the heat, cover the pot, and let them sit for an hour.

Directions (next day)

1. Add eight cups of water to a pot with beans. Boil. Lower to simmer, and cook the beans for thirty minutes.
2. As the beans simmer, start cooking the brown rice according to package directions (normally forty-five to fifty minutes for brown rice).
3. Add the remaining ingredients (except for the rice) to the beans and cook for an additional thirty minutes on simmer, or until beans are tender to serve. (Add a cup of water at a time if you desire a thinner soup.)
4. Once beans and rice are all done, place rice in an individual dish. Place bean soup on top of rice. Serve.

DAY 16

soar uphill!

Life isn't always a stroll. Sometimes it's hard to be alone; our stress levels rise; our heart beats out of our chest because we're so pressed down. We may feel as though the struggle will never end or we'll never get out from under the rain cloud. We become consumed by the drama.

I'm not going to deny that life can place great burdens on us. In such circumstances, my advice is to recognize that the drama is an external force and not let it live inside us. We should see any difficulty not as a battle or an uphill struggle, but something to make us tougher mentally, physically, and spiritually. That way, without us even realizing it, we're building a sturdy foundation, however messy the situation, so that when an even steeper hill comes our way, we'll soar up it! We'll be able to say to ourselves, "I am stronger. I am a survivor!" With an attitude of fortitude, our capacity for endurance will increase.

DRAMA-FREE MIND AND SPIRIT EXERCISES

Whether the hills are your family still not understanding and respecting your vegetarian choice, or something unrelated to vegetarianism, you may want to return to meat-based comfort food when you're under pressure. For some, every day will feel like an uphill climb, as you try your hardest not to eat meat. Say to yourself every minute and hour when the thought of meat arises: *I will soar uphill!* When you look back a year from now after being a vegetarian, you'll be able to affirm: "I felt as though I was beaten down, but I wasn't beaten. I didn't give up on myself, because I had the strength and endurance to soar uphill."

When hills arise on your vegetarian journey, I want you to tell yourself, as you climb them, *Soar uphill!* You'll look back and say, "I climbed that hill by gathering my endurance, strength, and everything I had in me. I *soared uphill!*" Soon enough, when you reflect on where you've been and where you're now going, you'll realize that it wasn't a hill you soared over, but a mountain!

DRAMA-FREE EXERCISE FOR THE BODY

Add spice to your exercise program by adding hills. Running up (and down) hills in your workout program will build more muscles and make you lean and sexy in those new jeans! Add intervals of hills in your walking, running, or biking. If you're going to the gym, a stair climber or treadmill can simulate hills. If you have stairs in your home, walk up and down for sixty seconds to five minutes a day. Hills are our friends. They always make us stronger.

energizing tortilla pinto bean wrap

LACTO-VEGETARIAN (WITH VEGAN OPTION)

When engaging in any exercise that's likely to deplete your stores of energy, a nutritious and fueling meal the night before is essential. You need energy to have the focus and strength to engage in your physical activity.

On one occasion, I planned to do a twelve-mile run, with no breaks for walking, in order to see what my body could do when I put my mind to it. Throughout the entire run, I felt incredibly relaxed. For almost two hours, I was lifted up on a cloud of peace, euphoria, and inspiration. In fact, I felt so great that I danced on my porch after the run to the last song on my music device before shutting it down and taking my dog for her walk. What provided me with the fuel I needed to surpass my goals? My meal from the previous evening: a vegetarian tortilla wrap.

In Christopher McDougall's *Born to Run: A Hidden Tribe, Super Athletes, and the Greatest Race the World Has Never Seen*, a coach notes that to be a strong runner you have to be a strong person. I truly believe that. I have my own formula: a vegetarian lifestyle = energy = fuel = going above and beyond = *I know I can!*

Cooking and Preparation Time: approximately 10 minutes
Servings: 1

Ingredients

1/4 cup of frozen corn

1/2 can pinto beans, drained and rinsed

1/8 tsp ground chipotle pepper (less, if milder version preferred)

1/8 tsp ground cumin

1/4 tsp cacao

1 flour tortilla

3 tbsp organic plain yogurt (vegan version: 3 tbsp vegan sour cream)

1 cup turnip greens, chopped roughly

2 slices of one tomato, cut in quarters

1/2 cup onions, sliced in strips

1/2 avocado, diced

Nutritional yeast, desired amount

Directions

1. In a microwave, heat corn, pinto beans, chipotle pepper, cumin, cacao, and 1 tbsp water in a small dish on *high* until corn is warmed, approximately 90 to 120 seconds.
2. Heat a tortilla until just warmed, not crisp in the oven or microwave.
3. Spread the yogurt or vegan sour cream on the tortilla.
4. Spread out the pinto beans, corn, and spice mixture (from step 1) on half of the tortilla.
5. Add the turnip greens, tomatoes, onions, and avocado on top of the beans and corn mixture. Sprinkle desired amount of nutritional yeast over tortilla stuffings.
6. Roll up the tortilla, and slice in half.
7. Plate and serve.

DAY 17

rewards of clear skin

You hear it over and over again from vegetarians: Once they began their lifestyle, their complexion improved. Within a month, the skin on their face became brighter, their acne or spots cleared up, their allergic reactions lessened, and their complexion became softer and younger-looking. If that's not sufficient enough reason to stay on your vegetarian journey, then think how much less money you'll have to spend on cosmetics and creams to cover up facial flaws. Once I became a vegetarian, my skin gradually developed a softness, smoothness, and brightness. I'd never had a problem with blemishes, but I was susceptible to an occasional allergic breakout depending on the time of year.

Within a month of becoming a vegetarian, not only did I no longer experience breakouts and my complexion brightened, but people at work saw that I had freckles on my nose! I'd known these people for six years, and they'd never noticed the freckles on my nose. It was as if they were

DRAMA-FREE MIND AND SPIRIT EXERCISES

1. Go makeup free on the weekends. It feels great to not be a slave to cosmetics! Your skin is naturally beautiful, and no enhancements are needed. Relax. This is your time!

2. Less is more. I wash my face with a basic soap, and apply a cocoa-butter lotion I've been using since I was a child. That's it! My face stays clear and free of blemishes. The more we apply to our skin, the more breakouts we have, because our pores become clogged or our skin reacts to the many chemicals in beauty products.

3. Try organic cosmetics, and products not tested on animals. Both are good for you, the animals, and the environment.

4. Try using just eye shadow, lip gloss, and mascara if you want to be *almost* makeup free. You'll have no dramatic late-for-work episodes, and you won't be trying to apply makeup as you drive to work or sit on the subway.

5. Did you know that cosmetic foundations actually remain on the skin even though you think you washed them off? Think twice when you reach for your foundation. Even out your skin with a vegetarian lifestyle based on whole foods: that is the best cosmetic foundation.

looking at me for the first time. I also stopped wearing makeup foundation—allowing the natural oils and water in my skin to assume that role. In fact, my skin was so clear that new arrivals at work thought I was only in my late twenties. They couldn't believe it when they discovered I was in my midforties.

It's not only the skin on your face that will brighten up and become smoother. The skin is the body's largest organ and it makes sense that a healthy, vegetarian lifestyle will help all your organs operate at their best, just as an unhealthful diet will cause all the organs to become dis-

DRAMA-FREE EXERCISE FOR THE BODY

Exercise and water are keys to clearer skin. Keep fueled during your exercise program by drinking water. Electrolyte-filled drinks are good for maintaining energy, but why not just go for the water to cleanse and replenish the body as you perspire? Electrolyte-filled drinks upset some people's stomachs. Drink lots of water during and after your exercise to stay hydrated, and for clear skin. Carry a handheld water bottle or camelback water holder. Some water bottles attach to their own Velcro belt, which you can wear on your hips when you walk, run, bike, or go to the gym.

eased. While it is indeed possible to be a "junk-food vegetarian," this book is premised on the fact that you're adopting a *healthful vegetarian lifestyle*. That means drinking water and not soda—which is full of sugars, chemicals, and even carcinogens (in some). Soda is not natural. Just think "natural" when you eat and drink.

Clearer skin is the result of drinking plenty of water and eating a variety of vegetables, fruits, whole grains, beans, and nuts in nutritiously prepared breakfasts, lunches, and dinners. Whole foods–based vegetarian meals heal the body naturally, as well as keep the skin fresh. For example, if I feel as though I'm becoming constipated or just want to keep my colon cleansed naturally without taking products, I prepare a dinner of sautéed beets with garlic in olive oil on a bed of wheat spaghetti; or I have a lunch of beet hummus. You won't need to stay by a bathroom when eating beets, or take magic pills and herbs or take a day or two off from work, or spend your whole weekend preparing yourself: the beets just work their way through the system naturally to clean out the colon and keep it healthy. The benefits of a healthy colon also include blemish-free skin.

If you're not a beets person, no problem. Turnip roots and okra also provide similar benefits to the colon. Simply cook up the okra and turnip roots into any dish. Remember not to overcook your vegetables, so that the nutrients remain. You'll have healthy skin and a well-functioning body.

water as i rise

VEGAN

Water is the fountain of youth—not only for making one's skin clearer, reducing body fat, and maintaining weight—but it has been documented to be a cure for many ailments. Studies in Japan and elsewhere have demonstrated that drinking a liter of water each morning before anything else is consumed can cure constipation, menstrual problems, arthritis, headache, asthma, vomiting, and gastritis, among other conditions. Water stimulates the production of fresh blood in the colon and activates the mucous therein, allowing the colon to flush itself more efficiently. Many, such as myself, who've integrated drinking a liter of water upon rising, have experienced frequent bowel movements where constipation may have been a problem in the past. Not only is my skin clearer but I no longer experience the stomach pains (and sounds) I once had after I ate meals. Drink your liter of water in the morning, and don't forget to continue to carry water with you in an aluminum type BPA-free drinking container throughout the day. Let water be your fountain of youth!

Preparation Time: None
Servings: 1

Ingredients

1 liter water, preferably natural spring water (approximately four-and-a-quarter measuring cups of water)

Directions

Many water therapies suggest drinking four cups to a liter of water upon rising from bed. The instructions also indicate that nothing should be eaten before the water is consumed, and to wait an hour before eating or drinking anything else. This is up to you. I drink a liter of water first thing in the morning, and then prepare my breakfast. Drink up for better well-being and health.

DAY 18

vegetarianism offers fuel for the body

We're now more than halfway through the month. We've touched on whole-foods vegetarian eating, and drinking water as a means of acquiring clear skin; detoxifying the body; and maintaining a healthy, functioning colon. We've explored the benefits of an active lifestyle and the importance of a strong mind to keep you on the path and not get sidetracked by the negativity and drama that may come your way.

Of course, at their most basic, food and water are fuel for the body's needs. If you're like me, when you ate meat you felt tired and sluggish afterward. It was sometimes hard to summon up the energy to exercise and you were exhausted and out of breath within fifteen minutes. The vegetarian diet provides you with natural energy that enables you not

DRAMA-FREE MIND AND SPIRIT EXERCISES

1. Plan your meals. Try making a large meal on Saturday or Sunday, and freeze the remainder to eat after work during the rest of the week. I like to make stews every Sunday and freeze what's left in individual serving proportions to eat over the next few weeks.

2. If you're cooking a lengthy meal on the weekend and freezing what's left, make quick twenty- to thirty-minute meals during the week (such as canned beans with fresh or frozen vegetables), if you're not heating up what you made on the weekend. Spice them up with a curry sauce, which takes only five to ten minutes to make.

3. Don't forget spaghetti. If you exercise (as I hope you do for your overall health), you need the carbohydrates for energy before the next day's workout. Whole-wheat spaghetti served with sautéed vegetables and garlic drizzled with olive oil adds a twist on the usual spaghetti and pasta sauce.

4. Fuel your body the night before your morning workout with a dinner that concentrates on replenishing your body with protein, complex carbs, or both. Your lunches should also provide fuel for the workday, and for your exercise routines, which may consist of the gym, walks, or runs. Try hummus wraps for lunches. Chickpeas are a great source of protein and energy. (Remember: you can use wraps of collard greens in lieu of flat bread or tortillas.) Stuff your wrap with greens (kale, mustard, turnips) for more nutrients, rather than lettuce. Include tomatoes, cucumbers, and onions. Add a healthful dip of salad dressing, raita (an Indian condiment made from mint, cucumber, and yogurt or), vegan sour cream, or tofu sauce.

to feel winded after walking upstairs, as I experienced before becoming a vegetarian.

As a runner, a hiker, and a backpacker, I provide fuel for my body not through pills but healthful carbohydrates, leafy greens such as mustard greens for clearer lungs, and a protein meal of curry, and Mexican and

African stews. After long runs and returning from long hikes, I avoid junk food and fast-food, and fuel my body again with meals cooked in Sister's kitchen.

Several Olympic champions and athletes have achieved their success on a plant-based diet. Ten-time gold-medal-winner Carl Lewis and world-record-holding ultramarathoner Scott Jurek are vegetarian and vegan, respectively. Baseball player Prince Fielder, renowned tennis players Billie Jean King and Martina Navratilova, basketball hall of famer Robert Parrish, football great Tony Gonzalez, and many others have either switched to a vegetarian lifestyle for better performance or were vegetarians starting out in their athletic career.

You don't need to pop pills, take muscle-building powders, or ingest other performance-enhancing products sold in stores to achieve optimal fitness. You can provide your body with protein and muscle-building fuel by eating whole-foods vegetarian meals. In addition to mustard greens helping me to breathe more easily, beans provide me with iron and protein to replenish my muscles, and vegetables and grains give me all the nutrients and energy I need to keep my body functioning well.

You can ignore the myth that vegetarians don't get enough protein and iron. We not only get a sufficient amount of protein and iron from our diets, but we actually ingest *more* protein than meat eaters because the protein from a plant-based diet is absorbed more efficiently than protein found in meat.

fuel me kushari

VEGAN

Fuel, repair, and replenish your overworked muscles with a traditional Egyptian meal: kushari. Kushari is an inexpensive dish that's sometimes known as the "fast food" of Egypt because you can enjoy this meal at virtually any restaurant, cafe, or street vendor. Kushari derives its "fast food" nickname not because it's packed full of junk calories, but because it's easy and quick to prepare. In addition, leftovers can be frozen easily, which makes it great for families on a budget. As one Egyptian on an episode of Anthony Bourdain's Food Network show *No Reservations* said, to indicate the importance of this traditional meal in Egyptian culture, "I would never marry an Egyptian woman who did not know how to cook kushari!"

Kushari is filling and packed with proteins, iron, and complex carbs. I love having this meal the day before a big run, long hike, or backpacking trip because it gives me sufficient energy to perform with endurance and it replenishes the muscles after a hard workout on the same day. Just as we shouldn't be waylaid by the protein myth, don't be afraid of carbs! We need complex—not simple—carbs to repair muscles, renew our cells, and give us the endurance to go the distance, whether we're exercising or working a long day.

Cooking and Preparation Time: approximately 45–50 minutes
Servings: 4

Ingredients

3 cups of wheat penne, spiral,
   or pasta of choice

1 cup of lentils, cleaned

1 cup of brown rice

3 cups water

4 medium garlic cloves, minced

Extra virgin olive oil

26-oz. jar roasted garlic pasta
   sauce

1 tsp cumin

1 tsp turmeric

1 tsp allspice

1/2 tsp hot pepper flakes or to
   taste

1/2 tsp ground chipotle powder
   or to taste

2 onions, halved and sliced

2 15-oz. cans chickpeas,
   drained

(*Optional:* Mexican style chipotle hot sauce)

Directions

1. Cook pasta according to package directions, drain, and set aside.
2. Cook lentils and rice together in three cups of water for forty-five to fifty minutes, until done. The lentils will be ready at the same time as the rice. Set aside when done.
3. Sauté garlic in 1 tbsp olive oil. Add pasta sauce, cumin, turmeric, allspice, hot pepper flakes, and chipotle powder. Heat all the way through. Set aside.
4. Cook onions in 2–3 tbsp olive oil until browned and a little crisp. Set aside.
5. Ready to serve: Place half to one cup of pasta in individual serving bowls.

6. Add the lentil and rice mixture on top of the pasta.
7. Place a quarter to half a cup of chickpeas on top of the rice and lentils.
8. Pour desired amount of pasta sauce on top of everything in bowl.
9. Add desired amount of crispy onions on top of everything.
10. Add extra Mexican-style chipotle hot sauce if preferred. (In Egypt, additional hot sauce is on the table when kushari is served in restaurants.)

DAY 19

step outside the box

As the old saying goes, "Each day is a new opportunity to start again." Each day brings forth a chance to discover more about yourself, to examine your mistakes from the day before and do things differently, and challenge yourself.

Vegetarianism opens an entire planet of unlimited possibilities that don't require any plane ticket or extra money to discover. Through your food choices, you'll travel to India, Pakistan, Ethiopia, Egypt, Morocco, Italy, Greece, Mexico, Peru, and a host of other countries that have vegetarian cuisine. Many of these countries' meals can be cooked in thirty minutes or less, which only gives you more reason to step outside the box to discover this whole new world.

You can explore new behaviors and do away with old patterns that never worked for you, and previously gave you health problems. You can participate in activities you were too fearful of trying before, or cooking gourmet meals you've always dreamed of, but lacked confidence to try.

DRAMA-FREE MIND AND SPIRIT EXERCISES

1. A good way to learn about another country's vegetarian recipes is through a cookbook that highlights that country's cuisine. If a recipe is meat-based, you can easily substitute meaty-type vegetables such as eggplant and portobello mushrooms. Or, you can try vegetarian meat substitutes such as tofu or seitan (wheat gluten). I love using eggplant or mushrooms instead of tofu or seitan: in my opinion, portobello mushrooms and eggplants absorb the flavors of the dish more quickly than either meat substitute. Furthermore, in many recipes, these two vegetables tend to be staples already.

2. In finding recipes from other countries to add variety to your vegetarian meals—rather than trying to turn the same old traditional SAD-based meals vegetarian, don't forget to find out how to use the many spices from each country. Did you know that cumin and curry aren't only popular in Indian food, but also in Mexican cuisine? Experiment with these spices; learn about how each one tastes and how it compliments the food. This information is always available in the front or back of each country's recipe book, or on the Internet.

3. Take a vegetarian cooking class. Many local cultural centers and farmers' markets now offer inexpensive classes where you can learn a wide variety of ways to cook vegetarian food.

4. Don't forget Sister's various world recipes after each day's motivation and on Sister's blog: www.sistervegetarian.com.

You can start an exercise program, or begin a different one. By investing your emotional, physical, and material resources in your new life, you'll receive tenfold back in well-being and success. You'll find yourself opening up and finding out things about yourself that you never knew existed. You'll stop being afraid and learn to enjoy the possibilities.

By taking each day as if it's a new beginning, and enjoying it to its fullest, you surround yourself with love—including enjoyment of who you are. You find yourself changing—internally and externally—before your eyes. You shed the hard shell of shyness and defeatism. You become "hip" to yourself and others, because you see fear as a four-letter word and that you're living out your dream. You discover that others want to know your secret of joy, how you live your day, how you exercise, and what recipes you use. In the words of poet Nikki Giovanni, "I am so hip even my errors are correct." Double-snap and nod!

DRAMA-FREE EXERCISE FOR THE BODY

Step outside the box in your exercise program and try something new—something you thought you may have been too old or out of shape to attempt. Register for races. It's fun! Start backpacking. I backpacked for the first time in my life at age forty-three. I slept in the wilds of the southern Appalachian regions of North Carolina with my husband and dog. I loved it, and haven't stopped since. When I stepped outside the box, my fears dissipated and I became a strong person—someone who said, "I *know* I can" rather than "I *think* that *maybe* I can."

Being a vegetarian taught me that by starting this journey alone without help or support, I was stronger than I thought I was. By taking a chance, I began to grow. I began to discover who I was rather than what someone else wanted me to be. It was up to me to decide if I wanted to continue to grow, or remain the same. I'll see you at the start line or wave hello as we backpack up the mountain!

sweet potato french fries

VEGAN

I love French fries with my delicious Cuban vegetarian sandwiches, veggie burgers, or vegetable wraps. French fries are vegan and can be nutritious, depending on how they're cooked. You should be careful, because many fries in frozen packets or restaurants may have been cooked in animal fat. To ensure your fries are healthful and fresh, make your own. I love to make fries not solely from the usual potatoes but from sweet potatoes or beets. How about turnip roots? Be creative and think outside the box for a nutritious and delicious accompaniment to your meals.

Cooking Time: approximately 30–40 minutes
Servings: 1–2

Ingredients

1 large sweet potato, washed (do not peel)

Extra virgin olive oil

Ground chipotle pepper

Smoked paprika

Black pepper

Garlic salt

(*Alternative*: in place of sweet potatoes, use sliced beets, sliced turnips, or make a medley of various vegetable fries.)

Directions

1. Preheat oven to 450 degrees F.
2. Slice sweet potatoes in one-inch slices (leave skin on for extra nutrients).
3. Place sweet potatoes on bowl, and drizzle lightly with extra virgin olive oil.
4. Lightly oil a pan with extra virgin olive oil.
5. Place sweet potato slices on oiled pan.
6. Season as desired with ground chipotle pepper, smoked paprika, black pepper, and garlic salt.
7. Place in oven and bake fifteen to twenty minutes on one side.
8. Turn over, and bake fifteen to twenty minutes until crisp on the other side.
9. Take out of oven and serve.

DAY 20

cooking like the pros

If preparing a vegetarian meal still seems like hard work to you, if you open your refrigerator and can't find anything to eat, if you feel that vegetarian meals are boring, or if you just don't feel like cooking and go to a fast-food chain for a double-stacked burger and fries . . . then you need to lighten up. Smile! Cooking vegetarian meals should be fun and easy. Preparing the meals and eating them should compliment your life, and not create drama.

Throughout this book, I've provided recipes that help you open your eyes to a world of meals; but I may have overlooked the key ingredient to every meal preparation: *have fun!*

A vegetarian lifestyle and meal preparation should be enjoyable, easy, and a great way to share laughter and good times with family and friends. If you find yourself bored with the recipes, then look at non-vegetarian recipes and turn them into vegetarian meals. You don't need to stick just with vegetarian cookbooks; an entire planet of dishes is waiting for you to enjoy while creating them. Throw a vegetarian party and cook like the pros!

Cooking entertaining meals for more than yourself and your family gets you through the drama of not knowing what to eat on a daily basis, and also entices others to try vegetarian meals. Your love of cooking shines in your meals, because you believe in the meals you prepared with love and congeniality. After you've found recipes you love, try them out on friends and family at a picnic, sit-down no-frills dinner, Sunday lunch buffet, Saturday college football gathering, or Sunday NFL football gathering. Be the celebrity chef for a day. Print the main recipe on index cards or amusing paper. Leave the recipe cards on the table next to the dish for others to take home and try on their own. Add fun drinks to compliment the meals. Eat, laugh, share food in love and delight in the company of family and friends.

My favorite TV chefs are those who combine real life and real food with gleeful meal preparations. You can see the twinkle in their eyes, and a love for the food. Although they're not vegetarians, two of my favorite

DRAMA-FREE MIND AND SPIRIT EXERCISES

Continue to motivate yourself through meal planning around themes. It's enjoyable and doesn't need to be time consuming. Play music from Africa, Mexico, India, or whatever region you cooked from that night. Even when heating up meals that I stored in the freezer, I still produce a themed meal, even if it's only for me. Every meal is distinctive because it's a way that you give love back to yourself. Remember: even if you're eating alone, you're always special. If my husband is working late, I light candles for myself, prepare a placemat with a cloth napkin, pour myself a glass of wine, and celebrate myself. Make your meal a daily, special event.

celebrity chefs are Bobby Flay and Rachel Ray because they're down-to-earth in their cooking techniques and make meals that can easily be prepared at home. I've decided that the key to cooking like the pros is threefold:

- Use what you have in your refrigerator and pantry, and substitute the recipe items you don't have with those you do, as you see fit.
- Make meals that are straightforward, which you can enjoy on different occasions.
- Center meals around family and friends, coming together to share in laughter and conversation. Food is a medium of communication.

DRAMA-FREE EXERCISE FOR THE BODY

The great thing about exercise is that, even if you indulge yourself at dinner the night before, exercise will burn the calories the next day. Tell me that isn't a drama-free incentive to exercise!

Of course, you can also have fun by challenging yourself to make elaborate meals. But even these don't have to take several hours to prepare. Some fancy feasts take only thirty minutes to an hour from start to finish.

You can also turn your exercise regimen into a chance for a gathering. Before the 2010 New York City Marathon, Bobby Flay cooked "Marathon Fettuccine" with Deena Kastor, the American Olympic bronze medalist and record-breaking marathoner, to showcase meals that long-distance runners could eat quickly and for maximum energy. Like Bobby and Deena, you could cook a themed meal as a motivator when you get burned out on eating alone or preparing the same dishes. If you run races, a pre-race party the night or two before might be a great motivator for you and your fellow competitors. Cook one or several pasta dishes for family and friends who'll also be running, or cheering you on as spectators. It's a great way to say "thank you" to the spectators and supporters running alongside you.

cooking like the pros fusion pad thai

VEGAN

Cooking like a pro involves using what you have to make an inexpensive meal, and have that meal turn out as though you should have your own show on the Food Network. I was "jonesing" for an Asian dish and hadn't yet done my weekly shopping. I also wanted something in thirty minutes or less. I did a quick inventory of my refrigerator and pantry, and got to work. I used wheat spaghetti to simulate Asian noodles, and added beet greens and other ingredients to create a Pad Thai recipe, based on a meal I'd had a couple of months previously in an Asian restaurant. The result is this awesome Fusion Pad Thai dish, created on the spot and on a budget! As it turned out, the dish tasted better than processed Pad Thai versions, and in my humble opinion better than some restaurant versions. I hope you enjoy this creative meal that lets you cook like a pro with what's on hand.

Cooking and Preparation Time: approximately 30 minutes
Servings: 4

Ingredients

Spicy Peanut Sauce Ingredients

5 tbsp organic peanut butter

3 tbsp organic brown sugar

4 tbsp Bragg's Liquid Aminos

1/2 tsp ground chipotle pepper

1 tsp minced garlic or 1 tsp ground garlic powder

2 tbsp water

3 tbsp Asian sweet chili sauce (alternative: sweet and sour sauce, mixed with a few drops of hot pepper sauce)

Noodles and Vegetables Ingredients

1/2 of 16-oz. box of wheat spaghetti (noodles broken in half) or 8-oz. box (noodles broken in half)

1/2 of 16-oz. frozen bag of stir-fry red and/or yellow peppers and onions

1/2 of 16-oz. bag of frozen French string beans

3 beet leaves chopped, roughly

3 beet stems cut in two-inch pieces

Spicy peanut sauce (recipe above)

1 cup peanuts

Directions

1. For the spicy peanut sauce, mix all the ingredients together until smooth and set aside.
2. Boil four cups of water.

3. Add all the Pad Thai ingredients above, except the spicy peanut sauce and peanuts. Cook for eight to ten minutes.

4. Drain pasta.

5. Return Pad Thai ingredients to pot. Add the spicy peanut sauce and peanuts.

6. Heat on low until warm.

7. Plate. Serve with chopsticks instead of forks, which I love to have around to use for Asian dishes in order to create an authentic atmosphere.

DAY 21

three weeks of drama-free vegetarian living: praise yourself!

Y*ou're feeling so alive right now! You go,* _____ [fill in your name]! You've completed three weeks as a vegetarian and your body feels renewed. If you don't think so, then remember how you felt before you started this journey. I'll bet you felt slow, sluggish, sick, worn-out, and worn down.

You're now a new person. Each day brings hope. You're strong and getting stronger. You're healthier than you were three weeks ago. You're a beautiful/handsome woman/man with clear skin that keeps getting clearer and brighter. You're exercising with vigor and are energetic. You're like a gazelle climbing upstairs, and an eagle soaring up hills.

The will to keep on this path is strong. You are *victorious*! You may have suffered defeat in some parts of this journey, but you crawled out of the well of discontent, you dusted yourself off, and got right back up and kept walking . . . kept climbing . . . and you weren't defeated. You can apply the words of Zora Neale Hurston to yourself: "I have been in Sorrow's kitchen and licked out all the pots. Then I have stood on the peaky mountain wrapped in rainbows, with a harp and sword in my hands." That's what I'm talking about!

You go, _____ [fill in your name] *with your bad self!*

Do you know how awesomely "bad" you can be at Day 21? Well, my Day 21 came around Thanksgiving. I faced the drama and challenges head-on and came out a winner. I decided that to avoid at least one aspect of the Thanksgiving drama—the eating of the turkey—I'd make and bring my own meal, for myself and others to enjoy. I made sure to let the cook know that I was a vegetarian, and that I was going to help her out by preparing another dish so that she wouldn't have to. (Preparing Thanksgiving meals can be stressful enough when you have to cook for ten or twenty instead of two or four people.) In my experience, when you bring your own vegetarian meal to a dinner surrounded

DRAMA-FREE MIND AND SPIRIT EXERCISES

Record your progress in a journal. Think about how you felt three weeks ago, before this journey started, and how you feel right now. Record how your health has become better, and how you're discovering new things about yourself. This is your wealth. Money comes and goes. It may buy you things to make you temporarily happy. But only one thing can make you truly content: a healthy mind, body, and spirit. Your health and well-being make you the strong person you are today. Health and well-being can remain and get better through this vegetarian lifestyle. You're a wealthy individual right now, and it just keeps getting better.

DRAMA-FREE EXERCISE FOR THE BODY

Record your progress in your exercise program. How did you feel three weeks ago? Were you out of breath within five, ten, or fifteen minutes? Can you now run, walk, bike, hike, or exercise for thirty minutes without feeling tired and out of breath? Are you exercising for longer periods of time on a weekly basis? What a motivation this is to know that you've built endurance! You're stronger than three weeks ago through your exercise program! Good job.

by meat eaters, you give them a chance to eat a dish they may not have considered either suitable for the holiday or full of taste and celebration.

Of course, your vegetarian dish may also break the ice and allow people to talk about whatever they may have been thinking about vegetarians or vegetarian dishes. How you handle what they say is up to you. You'll probably be asked the infamous question of why you became a vegetarian—especially when, as I did, you did so three weeks before Thanksgiving! I responded by saying that there was no better time for me to take back my health, since illness waited for no one and always took prisoners, so that I'd decided to act now for my benefit.

Now, some of you might think I'd put my foot in my mouth and was creating drama. But I remained true to myself, kept calm, and spoke without raising my voice in order to get my point across. As I did so, I felt I'd crossed a threshold of confidence in myself. I felt that I truly knew that my choice to become a vegetarian was not only the *correct* path for me, but that others should also seriously consider doing the same. My confidence was such that, by the end of Thanksgiving Day, I wasn't fending off hostile pseudo-questions but answering individuals who were genuinely interested in learning about the benefits of my lifestyle.

This behavior is being your "baddest" self. When we believe and have faith that our decision to adopt this lifestyle is correct, our confidence manifests itself in our thoughts, actions, and speech. I resisted the temptation and pressure to eat meat, and I survived the negative comments and aggressive questions—and I'm here to tell you that you can do the same. Not only have you survived twenty-one days, but you can survive twenty-one more, and then another twenty-one after that, and so on.

DRAMA-FREE EASY RECIPE

celebration grilled acorn squash salad

LACTO-OVO VEGETARIAN (WITH VEGAN OPTION)

Acorn squash has a beautiful, nutty, and buttery taste that I sampled raw as I peeled and chopped it into cubes for this recipe, and which it retains when cooked. I've never met a vegetable I didn't like, but acorn squash has to be number one on my list of the best tasting! I thought of this dish as a celebration of three weeks of success, because beautiful salads such as this one are usually reserved for get-togethers and picnics. I see completing three weeks of a vegetarian lifestyle as a party with family, friends, or just yourself. Turn on the music and dance! This is your picnic. This is your celebration.

Cooking and Preparation Time: approximately 16–20 minutes
Servings: 4–6

Ingredients

1 12-oz. package of spiral quinoa pasta

Extra virgin olive oil

1 medium acorn squash, about 1 lb. (peeled, and cut in cubes)

1 medium red bell pepper cut in strips, or three-quarters of a cup of roasted bell peppers from a jar cut in strips

Vegan liquid smoke

1/2 of medium onion, diced

(*Optional:* 1/2 tsp mesquite seasoning)

1/4 cup of sun-dried tomatoes, diced

2 small tomatoes cut in eighths

Mayonnaise (use vegan mayonnaise to make this a vegan meal)

Sea salt to taste

Black pepper to taste

Raw turnip leaves (washed) to serve as a bed for serving the pasta salad

Directions

1. Cook pasta according to directions. Drain and rinse with cool water. Set aside.

2. Set oven on broil. Lightly oil a cookie sheet with olive oil. Add acorn squash. If using fresh bell peppers, add this to cookie sheet. Drizzle acorn squash and bell peppers with liquid smoke. Broil for eight minutes on each side or until browned. Set aside when done.

3. Combine and mix in a large bowl quinoa pasta, acorn squash, bell peppers, onions, sun-dried tomatoes, tomatoes, mayonnaise or

vegan mayonnaise, sea salt, black pepper, and mesquite seasoning (*optional*).

4. Place a good amount of turnip leaves on each plate. Place pasta salad on top of the bed of leaves.

5. *Optional:* Serve with warmed, crusty Italian Tuscan-style bread drizzled with olive oil and topped with garlic slices, fresh basil (or turnip leaves), and sun-dried tomatoes.

DAY 22

be a child again

I've already mentioned how important it is to have a strong mind and to have fun. Now we need to chill out! I'm as bad as anyone, but I've noticed that many of us don't make it to our vegetarian or vegan goals because we're too hard on ourselves. That's drama right there! When we're hard on ourselves, we create a zone of negativity that surrounds us from when we wake up in the morning until we fall asleep at night. In fact, that negativity continues even as we sleep, just waiting for us to awake and repeat over and over again in our minds what we can't do, can't achieve, or can't maintain.

To penetrate the zone of negativity, we need to have the mind-set of a child. We need to be carefree and free-spirited. As adults we tend to overthink everything. We need to stop dwelling so much on the do's and don'ts of vegetarianism, making up rules that are hard to follow and that make us likely to fail before we even start. A child is always open to possibilities and enjoys life's little pleasures. She or he is enthusiastic about trying new things and likes to experiment. We, too, can do the same. Release all the chips on your shoulder about what you *should* do, and have fun playing. Don't beat yourself up if you can't afford organic or nongenetically modified produce, or if you can't eat seasonally or locally, or if you aren't eating raw food every day or dining on exotic fruits for breakfast. Do what you can with what you have.

Another aspect of childhood is that the more rules you impose on kids, the more likely they are to rebel. It's the same with your vegetarian journey: the more strictures you have at the start, the more your psyche is going to resist. For all the rules and regulations that vegetarians like to impose on themselves and others, the best way to get someone on your side is to show them how easy the diet is, and then let them gradually go where they need to go from there. So stop the rules. Stop creating drama that doesn't need to exist. We have enough drama already with our jobs, bills, and balancing family and work life! Enough! Chill out!

DRAMA-FREE MIND AND SPIRIT EXERCISES

1. Repeat to yourself: *Be like a child.*
2. Write down why you started this vegetarian journey as a reminder to yourself to relax. When vegetarians or vegans come up to you and tell you what and what not to eat, remember who you are and how far you've come on the journey. Each person's journey is different, so what may work for them may not for you. Don't feel as though you haven't been on the right path. You *are* on the *right path.* Certainly be open to their ideas, and change if you want to, but don't be hard on yourself and don't let them be hard on you. Thank them for the advice, and, as the Buddhists say, "Take from it what you want and apply it to your life."

DRAMA-FREE EXERCISE FOR THE BODY

1. You can carry your childlike disposition into your exercise program. Don't punish yourself for not working out rigorously enough or not seeing the results you want immediately. Simply starting an exercise program will bring its own rewards. Children love to move, dance, skip, hop, and run; they do it spontaneously as expressions of their joy at living. For instance, I love to run or hike in the rain, without an umbrella. Why do we love to run and play in the rain when we're children, but run for an umbrella as an adult? Rain won't make us sick; a compromised immune system does. Being vegetarian fortifies our immune system. Play, walk, and run in the rain. Unless it's thundering and lightning while raining, you'll be fine.

2. Another childlike exercise is to rake leaves and jump on the leaf pile. I love raking leaves, because I'm reminded of when I was a child in New Jersey. An added benefit is that raking leaves burns more calories (and is a lot quieter and more environmentally friendly) than using a leaf blower.

3. How about roller-skating? I loved roller-skating in the mid-1970s. I had pink pompoms on my skates. It's still fun as an adult.

4. Jump rope. According to the healthytimesblog.com, ten minutes of jumping rope at 120 revolutions per minute produces the same level of cardiovascular fitness as running one mile in ten minutes.

5. Join an adult league in softball, bowling, basketball, volleyball, dodge ball, or flag football suitable for your age group. It's actually more fun playing with your age group, as you have someone to laugh with about age-related aches or pains!

6. Remember to step out of the box with your exercise routine.

the child in me veggie burger

VEGAN

Eating a veggie burger reminds me of being carefree as a child with catsup and mustard slithering down the cracks of my mouth as I ate my mother's homemade burgers. As a vegetarian adult, I know the dangers of eating meat and the disease it can produce in one's body. However, there are so many versions of veggie burgers—the most popular being made with beans and rice—that you could probably eat a different burger each day for a year. I've decided to have some fun and make a veggie burger that's made of just that: *veggies*. I love using veggies for a burger: the crispiness of the burger's outside against the melody of moist vegetables inside combines on your palate to form . . . well, a merriment of delight. After all, it's child's play.

Cooking Time: approximately 16–20 minutes
Servings: makes 6–8 veggie burgers

Ingredients

2 cups fresh turnip roots, diced (washed and leave skin on). (*Note*: turnip roots have anti-oxidant and cancer-fighting properties.)

1 cup yellow squash, diced (washed and leave skin on)

1 cup carrots, diced (washed and leave skin on)

1 medium onion cut in quarters

4 garlic cloves

1 1/2 cups bulgur wheat

1/2 cup old-fashioned oatmeal

1 tsp vegan liquid smoke

1/2 cup cashews

1 cup of mustard leaves (leaves left whole)

1 tsp sea salt, or to taste

1 tsp ground black pepper, or to taste

Extra virgin olive oil

2 tbsp water (as needed to moisten mixture)

Topping

Cuban Aioli Sauce (see Day 5 recipe)

Wheat buns

Veggie Burger Directions

1. Preheat oven to 450 degrees F.
2. Mix in food processor all ingredients except Cuban Aioli Sauce and water. If the mixture seems a little dry after mixing, then add two tbsp water. Add more water if needed to get a moist but not watery mixture to form patties.
3. Lightly oil baking sheet with olive oil.

4. Form mixture into six to eight patties, and place on baking sheet.

5. Bake for ten minutes on each side for a total of twenty to thirty minutes, or until firm. Broil for additional two to three minutes for a crispy, outer topping.

6. Serve on a wheat bun with Cuban sauce, sliced tomatoes, and turnip leaves topped on bun.

7. Side dish suggestions: Sweet Potato French Fries (Day 19) or Celebration Grilled Acorn Squash Salad (Day 21).

DAY 23

i am not afraid

"Grab the broom of anger and drive off the beast of fear."
—ZORA NEALE HURSTON

Throughout my journey as a vegetarian and then vegan, I've discovered my shyness and fear dissipating. To paraphrase Zora Neale Hurston, "I drove off the beast of fear." I have become more extrovert in crowds, and more willing to try something new. There's something about being a vegetarian that makes you look your fear in the eye, and scare it off.

Perhaps it was walking this journey without a support system; or developing determination to get right back up after eating meat again; or being in a minority at family gatherings or the only vegetarian at work or at holiday lunch parties; or feeling as though your path is invisible to others (as happened when I was given a meat-based cookbook for my birthday). All these have made me stronger. You too will develop your fearlessness.

I was once afraid to take a stand and speak out for what I believed in. I had to clear my mind of past fear and nervousness in order to move forward. I had to realize my fears and shyness were making me stagnant. Being a vegetarian has made me stronger—someone who stood up against cruelty to animals and in favor of a healthier life. I followed the words of Bob Marley, "Emancipate yourself from mental slavery. None but ourselves can free our minds."

Recently, I joined a demonstration in my city to protest the use of injured circus elephants. I knew there was a possibility I might be arrested if our peaceful demonstration went awry, but I put my fear aside and joined in. If I'd been the person I was before, I'd never have participated in the demonstration nor stood up against cruelty toward animals. As it turned out, my fears of being arrested were almost made real when the officials at the venue we were targeting asked the local police to take pictures of the twenty-

DRAMA-FREE MIND AND SPIRIT EXERCISES

1. As a gospel song says, "Be encouraged and encourage yourself." Encourage yourself by writing down how, in the past, the slightest little disturbance in your journeys (vegetarian and otherwise) made you feel like giving up.
2. Now write down how you feel when you become agitated. You'll realize that you've grown stronger and fearless. You can handle changes in your routine much better than you could a month ago.
3. Refer to this journal entry again and again for encouragement.
4. Add to the entry as you continue through the weeks, months, and years of your journey. You'll witness how you've grown.
5. Share your testimony with those who are beginning their vegetarian journey or considering it. This can also be their fuel for their endurance and strength.

five demonstrators, in case of any incidents. I held my STOP ANIMAL CRUELTY sign high with great pride. Despite provocation, we maintained a peaceful disposition as patrons drove into the parking lot. Fists were shaken in our face, but we continued to smile and even joked with the traffic policeman who served as our protection. I was proud to stand for something I believed in and knew was correct. I took a stand, and left fear behind.

The following Saturday, I attended a march—the first time I'd been to a march for anything! The occasion was a gathering on behalf of human rights, which my vegan action group had expanded from its initial forum for the rights of nonhuman animals. Our call was for a better nation and planet that respected the rights of humans *and* animals, an increased consciousness of the environment, and our need to protect all of them. (The march made the national news, and my friends and family called me to ask whether what they'd seen on television was the event I'd participated in.)

During the march, I lifted my ANIMAL RIGHTS banner high and walked proudly the two-plus miles route, which ended at the state capitol and legislative buildings. Members of my vegan action group had indicated to me that in past years onlookers had shouted threats and slurs because of the presence of an animal rights group at a human-rights march. I knew there was a chance this would happen again. Nonetheless, we walked tall and held our signs, and committed ourselves to the kind of peaceful witnessing that was the hallmark of Mahatma Gandhi's campaigns in South Africa and India. For the first time, I was told, our group experienced no problems. Perhaps the recognition that animal rights, vegetarianism for health and the environment, and the right of people to live in wellness and dignity is catching on. Whatever the reason, I was proud that day once more to make a stand. To no longer be afraid has been one of the most profound lessons of my becoming a vegetarian.

DRAMA-FREE EASY RECIPE

i'm not afraid calzone

LACTO-OVO VEGETARIAN (WITH VEGAN OPTION)

I once was afraid to make calzones. I loved to eat them, but was intimidated by the supposed intricacies involved in the process. Well, I don't fret anymore, and you shouldn't either! You can make this hearty meal in thirty to thirty-five minutes with the same love, warmth, and heartiness of the calzone stuffings you'd find in your favorite Italian restaurant. This meal uses ready-made refrigerated pizza dough, which cuts the cooking time to a meal in thirty minutes, after fifteen to twenty minutes of preparation.

Cooking and Preparation Time: approximately 30 minutes
Servings: 2

Ingredients

Extra virgin olive oil

1 large turnip root, diced
   (washed with skin left on)

2 Roma tomatoes, diced

4 slices of eggplant, chopped

1/2 cup sliced onions

2 tsp vegan liquid smoke

1 tsp Mexican chipotle pepper
   hot sauce

1 can nondairy refrigerated
   pizza dough

3 slices of fresh mozzarella
   cheese (vegan version: use
   vegan mozzarella cheese)

1/2 cup ricotta cheese (vegan
   version: use vegan cottage
   cheese)

Nutritional yeast

1/2 jar of marinara pasta sauce

Directions

1. Preheat oven to 375 degrees F.
2. Lightly oil pan with olive oil.
3. Marinate in bowl turnip roots, tomatoes, eggplant, and onions in liquid smoke and hot sauce.
4. Roll out pizza dough horizontally for approximately twelve inches in length on a cutting board.
5. Lightly brush olive oil on dough facing up.
6. Spread ricotta cheese or vegan cottage cheese on one half of dough.
7. Add mozzarella or vegan mozzarella slices on top of ricotta.
8. Add marinated vegetables on top of cheeses.
9. Sprinkle nutritional yeast on top of vegetables (use as desired).
10. Fold over other half of dough on top of stuffing and pinch ends to form a seal.

11. Lightly brush top with olive oil.
12. Place in oven and bake thirty minutes or until golden on top.
13. Remove from oven, slice in half.
14. Serve with a side-dipping bowl of marinara pasta sauce, warmed.

DAY 24 COMPLETED: _____

DAY 24

second chance at life

So much drama is created when we're trying to battle illnesses, and overcome the depression that surfaces as we suffer from those ailments. By now, you'll know the answer to preventing or reversing those conditions! Being a vegetarian gives you a second chance to get your blood pressure, diabetes, heart disease, colon cancer, high cholesterol, and other conditions in check—or better yet, remove illness from your system altogether. You walked away from meat to give yourself hope for a better tomorrow. You had to let that part—that love of meat—die to give yourself a second chance at life. You had to say *goodbye* to something you've known a long time (meat) in order to say *hello* to something better (better health through a vegetarian lifestyle). Some studies say that you can add seven years to your life by adopting a vegetarian diet. What an incentive to continue!

DRAMA-FREE MIND AND SPIRIT EXERCISES

Visit your physician for your annual checkups. This is your monitor system, especially if you have a history of heart disease and diabetes. Stay on top of how often you're checked up and for what conditions. You may start to visit the doctor much less, and your doctor may begin to remove you from medications. You may be paying out fewer co-pays for visits to the doctor's office and filling fewer prescriptions. Studies have shown that a vegan diet can reverse diabetes and heart disease, where people have gone from sixteen medications to only four. Give yourself a second chance at life!

DRAMA-FREE EXERCISE FOR THE BODY

Exercise lowers high blood pressure, keeps diabetes in check, and wards off many illnesses and cancers. Let this be your incentive and motivation to continue with your exercise program. If you haven't done so already, take your exercise program to the next level. Add weights, rope jumping, calisthenics, yoga, strength training—all these require little or no money. There's no excuse. Start today and go to the next level. You owe yourself a second chance.

DRAMA-FREE EASY RECIPE

second chance cold vegetable wrap

LACTO-VEGETARIAN (WITH VEGAN OPTION)

Eating vegetables raw rather than cooked allows them to retain more of their antioxidant and cancer-fighting power to heal our bodies. This wrap offers a quick meal for after work, lunchtime, or even as a picnic for two.

Preparation Time: approximately 10 minutes
Servings: 1

Ingredients

3 tbsp organic plain yogurt
(vegan version: 3 tbsp vegan
sour cream)

1 flour tortilla

3–4 large turnip leaves (Note:
turnip leaves are known
for their cancer-fighting
properties.)

1/2 cup chopped cucumbers
(cleaned and skin left on)

1/4 cup of onions, sliced

1 garlic clove, sliced

1/2 cup chopped tomatoes

Nutritional yeast to taste

Ground chipotle pepper to taste

Ground smoked paprika to taste

Directions

1. Spread yogurt or vegan sour cream on a tortilla.
2. Place on one half of the tortilla all the remaining ingredients.
3. Roll tortilla.
4. Slice in half.
5. Plate and serve.

DAY 25

breathe deep and relax

Studies have shown that vegetarians have lower levels of depression, and are happier and more relaxed. Wow! This is sufficient motivation for me. Keep me signed on *this* path! This is drama-free living!

A question I'm often asked is how I keep being a vegetarian in a world where meals of meat are ubiquitous. In some ways, this entire book is a response to that question. But the short answer is that I remain myself and try to relax! That's my advice to you, and I can't say it enough. This lifestyle should not be stressful. Remember when we talked about following your own path and not trying to be the vegetarian or vegan you don't want to be? That's still true. When we follow our own path, we stick with the plan. Relax and enjoy this vegetarian journey.

A central reason why it's important to learn how to relax as you walk the vegetarian path is that challenges will inevitably arise, often when we least expect them. These storms are not the same as the drama. We

DRAMA-FREE MIND AND SPIRIT EXERCISES

1. Write down whom you admire as a vegetarian or vegan.
2. Why do you admire that person (write their goals, actions, ideas, and whatever attracts you to how they lead this lifestyle)?
3. Write down your *own* goals, actions, ideas, what attracts you to a vegetarian or vegan lifestyle, what you plan to accomplish and get out of it.
4. Compare your list of goals with the person you admire. You'll find out that your list seems more significant than that of the person you admire because it's more tailored to you and your success as a vegetarian or vegan.
5. Write down how you plan to maintain this lifestyle—such as meal ideas, pantry grocery shopping list, exercise.
6. Post your list where it can be seen daily.
7. Honor your path.

create drama through our actions and reactions. Storms will come and blow over; but drama can last a lifetime if we don't handle it. No one said life would be easy; it's how we handle those dark moments that make the difference between sailing through the turbulent seas or sinking into the depths. What you need to understand is that *you* have the power to decide how to handle those situations.

Food is often a way that we respond to pressure. Perhaps in the past, food was a crutch, an anchor, or balm—you choose your metaphor—when trouble arose. You may have reached for the cheeseburgers, greasy fries, pepperoni pizzas, pints of ice cream, or sugar-loaded cookies to ease your stress. What you need to understand is that you are no longer the same person. You have the strength to calm the storm and lead a drama-free life. You have learned how to eat healthily. These lessons that you are living right now can allow you to relax and practice meditation for peace as the winds rock your boat.

For instance, the very week

that I signed the contract for this book, my father was diagnosed with pancreatic cancer. When the surgeon brought us into the room and told us that cancer cells were covering my father's pancreas, I was composed as I listened. What I heard was distressing, but I also knew that a higher power had control and that all I had to do was to remain calm. I didn't need to run to the hospital cafeteria to stuff my face with junk food, as I would once have done to comfort myself. Later that day, as I ate my vegan meal, I held fast to the knowledge that "this, too, will pass." I knew that, whatever the situation, I had to fuel my mind, body, and soul so I could remain strong and in the right frame of mind for my parents. I needed the focus and calmness to help my parents with shopping, appointments, and cleaning along with working my full-time job.

By being relaxed and at peace as the winds of life buffeted me, I believe that I opened up possibilities for healing. Since his diagnosis, my father has asked me more about how a vegetarian lifestyle might be beneficial to him. He has not yet returned to his athletic lifestyle of bicycling daily or going to the gym, as he had been doing at the age of seventy-three before the operation, but I have faith that everything is going to be all right.

When my father asked me how I kept being positive through his illness, I told him that I knew that, when we breathe and relax, we can

DRAMA-FREE EXERCISE FOR THE BODY

1. Don't forget to take a day or two off to relax from exercise. If you're a runner, you may want to rest on two consecutive days. Our muscles need time to heal and repair themselves. Injuries happen when we overuse our bodies because we don't rest them enough.
2. Enjoy those rest days with a good book, knitting, family time, friend time, or just doing nothing. Doing nothing can be a form of doing something when our bodies need replenishing.

maintain peace of mind that can handle any situation without drama. Breathe deeply through your vegetarian journey. Have a relaxed state of mind to continue on this vegetarian path with trust and faith. Everything will be all right.

breathe deep herbal ice tea

VEGAN

I love to relax at work or home with a hot cup of herbal tea. I love tea so much that I'm able to drink it in the summer. However, when it's ninety degrees or higher outside in North Carolina, a cooling and refreshing herbal ice tea is what I really need to unwind and enjoy the beauty of nature. This recipe is a twist on the green tea that can be found in any store. If green tea is not your preference, try other varieties of herbal and fruit teas for a refreshing session of breathing deeply, relaxing, and enjoying your meditative time. I pour my tea into a wine goblet, sit outside on my lawn chair, and relish a relaxing afternoon with nature. The wineglass signifies that it's okay to dress up! Every meal, even teatime, should be a special ceremony for you. This is all about you.

Cooking and Preparation Time: approximately 10 minutes
Servings: 1

Ingredients

Pomegranate berry green tea (or any variety of herbal tea you prefer)

Wine goblet or medium-sized wineglass

2 tsp agave

3 fresh mint leaves

6 ice cubes

Directions

1. Boil water in a kettle on the stove.
2. As the kettle is waiting to boil, put six ice cubes in a wine goblet rinsed with cold water and chill in the freezer.
3. Once the water is ready, place the teabag in a large mug and steep for five minutes.
4. Remove the tea bag.
5. Add agave into the brewed tea, stir, and pour in the chilled goblet.
6. Place fresh mint leaves in the goblet.
7. Serve. Ahhhhhhhhh! Refreshing, inspiring, and I'm breathing deeply to relax.

DAY 26 COMPLETED: _____

DAY 26

it all has to do with the individual journey

W e've already talked about how this journey is yours and no one else's. But let's go a little deeper. When I think of the individual journey, I'm reminded of socks.

I love to knit socks—mainly because they remind me of our lives. We're all born with DNA, which has the same structure for everyone. But contained in that DNA are instructions that form an intricate and unique knitted network that shapes who we are as individuals. In the same way, you can take a pattern for knitted socks and duplicate it many times—with millions of people knitting socks from the same pattern. However, no matter if one person knits from the same pattern a million times, or a million people knit from the same pattern once, each pair of socks will turn out differently.

Take it from me. I've knitted many socks using the same basic knit

166

DRAMA-FREE MIND AND SPIRIT EXERCISES

1. It's payback time! No, I'm not talking about revenge. I'm talking about paying back those who've kept you going on your vegetarian journey. Thank them. Give them a hug. Cook a special meal for them. Show them how much you appreciate their support. As the saying goes, "'Tis better to give than receive," and thus far we've been receiving their loving support. When we give back, that generosity comes back to us in many positive ways and rewards.

2. It's also pay it forward time! That means, when someone gives you something positive, give that something to somebody else. You've probably already started to spark the curiosity about your new lifestyle in a lot of people. They're seeing so many positive changes in your life that they want to know your secret to success. My advice is to give supportive words of wisdom. Think about how full that person's spirit will feel when filled with words of love and encouragement from a fellow vegetarian.

pattern, and each time the socks take on a different personality of their own, whether I use the same or different types of yarn. They may have colorful stripes, intricate patterns, or bright and bold colors. I might have woven in pictures, provided different finishing touches, and more. Even if I consciously try not to deviate from the pattern, the socks still turn out differently each time—from the way the needles were held (tight, loose, or just firm enough). I may have been a little sleepy when I was knitting, or perhaps I was hyper alert; I may have been knitting outdoors or indoors, relaxed or tense—no pair is exactly the same.

That's how I see our different vegetarian journeys. You can look at it in two ways. One way is to say that we may look very different, but in the end we're all socks. Another way is to say that although we're all socks, we're all very different. Either way is true. From one perspective, we may be many different types of vegetarian—because we support animal rights, because we want to maintain our health, because we care about the environment, because we dislike the taste of meat, because it's part of our religious upbringing or beliefs (or some combination of all of the above)—but we're all on the same path.

From another perspective, we're all on the same path, even though we're following many different types of vegetarianism. I may like to cook at home; someone else may prefer to eat out. I may love food for its different flavors; someone else may see it only as fuel. Some may see veganism as only a diet; others may see it as a lifestyle that encompasses not using any animal products and making a commitment to living nonviolently.

Of course, we can change our mind when we're exposed to more information, but my larger point is that vegetarians shouldn't be fighting with one another to claim a higher moral ground. We don't need the drama, and we shouldn't judge others, for they may well turn around and judge you. None of us is perfect. We may not know the reasons why they haven't reached "our level." Perhaps they can't afford it yet; perhaps they're under enormous pressure to conform? Who wants to be considered a food snob?!

Instead, we should lift up our fellow sister and brother vegetarians, no matter what path they've chosen. Surely we could agree that, at the very least, we're all on a journey to take back our health and respect the environment. Why not provide encouragement rather than criticism, wisdom rather than polemics, and advice rather than judgment to guide others to make the best decisions for their own journey? Let us be champions of faith and positive reinforcement! Let us be role models.

Now that you've made it to Day 26, you can offer encouragement to others. Doing so uplifts you as well. When we uplift and encourage others, drama has no place in our lives. Words of wisdom go further than dictating what "should" and "should not" be done.

Friends are as companions on a journey, who ought
to aid each other to persevere in the road to a happier life.

—PYTHAGORAS

DRAMA-FREE EASY RECIPE

individual falafel journey

VEGAN

Falafel, a popular street food that originated in Egypt and is now widespread throughout the Middle East, is a fried ball or patty made from chickpeas and spices. Traditionally, falafel is served in a pita or wrapped in flat bread. The balls themselves are topped with lettuce, hot sauce, tahini sauce, tomatoes, pickled vegetables, or another condiment. They can also be eaten individually as an appetizer with a side dip of tahini sauce, peanut sauce, cucumber, or yogurt-mint sauce.

In this recipe, I oven-baked the falafel, since it was healthier than deep-frying them. This recipe makes approximately thirty-five balls. Falafel can also be used with whole-wheat spaghetti and marinara sauce to simulate spaghetti and meatballs. I also took a different tack in wrapping the falafel in a collard-green leaf, drizzled with a peanut sauce, with chopped kale on top. I've also wrapped falafel in a Mediterranean-style flat bread with turnip leaves, cucumbers, onions, and tomatoes. Mmmm good! Be creative with this meal.

Cooking and Preparation Time: approximately 40 minutes
Servings: 35 individual falafel balls
Storage: Falafel stores easily in an airtight container in the freezer. Defrost the individual balls, depending on how many you'd like to serve.

Ingredients

1-lb. bag of dried chickpeas, soaked overnight, drained, and rinsed

6 cloves of garlic crushed

1 large onion finely chopped

1 cup mustard greens, roughly chopped

1 tsp smoked paprika

1/2 tsp ground chipotle pepper

1 tsp ground coriander

2 tsp ground cumin

1 tsp ground curry powder

1 tsp garlic salt

1 small chili red pepper (deveined and seeds removed), diced fine

1 tsp baking soda dissolved in 1/2 cup water

Olive oil

Directions

1. Preheat oven to 375 degrees F.
2. In a food processor, grind chickpeas. Add all the remaining ingredients except the olive oil, and mix in the food processor.
3. Lightly oil cookie sheet pan with olive oil.
4. From the mixture form balls approximately one inch in diameter, and place on cookie sheet pan.
5. Bake fifteen minutes on each side, until golden brown.
6. Broil two to three minutes on each side for extra crispness.
7. Remove and serve as desired.

DAY 27

calling upon our life force

We create drama in our lives when we ignore our inner voice, which knows what's best for us, and don't energize our chi. The word "chi" means "life force" or "inner energy." Although chi comes from Chinese philosophical and religious traditions, many cultures have an equivalent. In the West African Yoruba tradition, it is known as *ashé*. The Ancient Egyptians called it *ka*. Native Americans name it the *Great Spirit*; Hawaiians term it *mana*. In Japan, chi is known as *ki*, and in India it is called *prana*, or "breath." Echoes of chi are found in the Hebrew *ruach* ("breath") and the Christian concept of the Holy Spirit. Whatever its name or root tradition, chi is a vital force that animates us and provides us with the energy that both fosters inner peace and connects us with the universe as a whole.

DRAMA-FREE MIND AND SPIRIT EXERCISES

1. Sit in a quiet room on the floor with your back straight, legs crossed in front of you, and hands either on your lap, clasped, or in a prayer position. Breathe through your nose and exhale through your mouth. Feel and hear your breath. You are becoming calm and peaceful.

2. Repeat a mantra, such as *I am victorious as a vegetarian*; *I am at peace*; *I can, I will, I am*; or any positive statement that reinforces positive chi within you.

3. Practice this for five to ten minutes in the morning and evening, or once a day when it's "your time," without interruption.

4. Write down how you feel before practicing this meditation to build upon your energy now and afterward. How do you feel afterward? Do you feel more focused as a vegetarian? More confident at maintaining a vegetarian lifestyle when others around you may be trying to persuade you otherwise? Do you feel more confident in general? If not, write down how you can change yourself to be more confident and find peace in this lifestyle. Meditate using your inner energy on what would work best for you to undertake this beautiful vegetarian journey.

5. Don't forget, chi works best with a smile. Smile inwardly and outwardly in everything you do. When we smile, things become simple and less stressful, and we realize what works best for us. We are at peace with ourselves and the world.

As a vegetarian, I see chi as the substance of our strength. Chi connects us with our conscience to take back our health and become stronger mentally, physically, and spiritually as we practice a vegetarian lifestyle. It helps us to build upon the belief that we can and will lead healthful vegetarian lives without others trying to sabotage us. Chi is what we can draw on to give us the confidence, motivation, and inspiration to be happy, strong, and at peace: to be and stay a vegetarian in the midst

DRAMA-FREE EXERCISE FOR THE BODY

Conjure up your chi in your exercise program. Meditate for at least five minutes before you exercise for focus and for strength. Meditate at least five minutes after exercising to wind down and center yourself. You'll feel more energized and focused on the path before you.

of the storm; to resist temptations to return to unhealthful lifestyles that involve meat and junk food; and to know when to step forward, when to wait, and when to climb.

Chi is the inner life force that makes us unique individuals—separating us from one another because we have our own inner energy to know what path is right for us. But it also joins us together as the universal energy force. If we learn to listen to our chi—that inner energy and the energy of the universe—we will go where we need to go, and know we're on the right path. Chi gives us hope when we feel hopeless and lack faith. To use the Christian tradition's notation: it is the substance of things hoped for and the evidence of things not seen.

Draw upon your life force. Speak to it; listen to it. When your mind, body, and spirit act in unison rather than work against each other, you'll be drawing the energy from within you and using it positively. Don't create drama in your life by listening to someone whose ideas contradict your determination and vision for a better life for yourself. Let chi turn your vegetarian journey into a stress-free, enjoyable, empowering, and committed one—full of life and zest.

i am chole palak

VEGAN

Chole Palak is a traditional Indian curry meal made with chickpeas and greens. Curry powder and turmeric are known in Indian medicine to have antioxidant, anti-inflammatory, and cancer-preventative qualities—benefits and healing properties that we're only just starting to learn about in the West. When we add these spices to meals on an ongoing basis, we increase our body's ability to fight ailments. Indeed, several studies have been conducted to determine whether these spices prevent Alzheimer's disease. Whatever their particular medicinal qualities, curry and turmeric provide spice and energy for our chi. This thirty-minute meal is delicious, nutritious, and healing.

Cooking Time: approximately 30 minutes
Servings: 4

Ingredients

3 tbsp olive oil

1 medium onion, minced

5 medium garlic cloves, minced

1 14 1/2-oz. can diced, roasted
　garlic tomatoes

2 cups of fresh mustard greens,
　chopped roughly

3 tbsp curry powder

1 tsp garam masala

1/2 tsp dry cilantro

1/2 tsp turmeric powder

1/2 tsp coriander powder

1/2 tsp cumin powder

1/2 tsp chili powder

2 15 1/2-oz. cans of chickpeas,
　drained

1/2 15 1/2-oz. can black
　beans, drained

1 cup of water

Directions

1. Heat olive oil in pan.
2. Add onions and garlic, and sauté for five minutes until pale in color.
3. Add tomatoes and sauté for one to two minutes.
4. Add mustard greens and all remaining spices. Sauté for five minutes.
5. Add chickpeas, black beans, and water.
6. Simmer for five minutes. Stir occasionally with a wooden spoon.
7. Plate and serve.

Serving Suggestions

1. *Breads:* Serve with warmed chapati bread, wheat tortilla, or pita bread with a side dish of vegan sour cream or plain yogurt. (In India, it's traditional to serve yogurt with curry as a coolant.)

2. *Rice or Grains:* Serve on top of a bed of brown rice, bulgur wheat, or couscous.

DAY 28

four weeks
of vegetarian living

Let's Get Our Praise Dance on Again
"If you know whence you came, there are absolutely
no limitations to where you can go."

—JAMES BALDWIN

You've now lived four weeks as a vegetarian! *You go!* You're amazing and a wonder to behold. Before you began your journey, you may have said to yourself that you couldn't do it. But you learned to believe in yourself and trust your decision. You said, "Yes I can!" And you did it! You believed it! You said "I will" and you made it happen! This is a time to celebrate and honor your accomplishments.

Spread the word! Tell others how good you feel as a vegetarian! Tell a meat eater! When you glow and show your praise inwardly, your inner peace and joy will show on the outside. You may influence someone to become a vegetarian just by your positive actions, smiles, and words. Dance. Dance. Dance. You deserve it! Let's get that praise dance on! *You are worthy to be praised!*

Four weeks is not just a number in a long journey; you're a better person. This period has strengthened you in areas you knew needed strengthening (and some you didn't). The Greek philosopher Heraclitus observed, "You can't step into the same river twice." In the same way, you're not the same vegetarian today as you were yesterday or you will be tomorrow. Every day we learn more about ourselves and grow on this journey. Some veteran vegetarians may feel as though they've no more room or areas for growth, but I don't believe that's true. As long as we're alive,

DRAMA-FREE MIND AND SPIRIT EXERCISES

Dancing is a great way to relieve stress. Many cultures use dance as a form of celebration in their daily rituals—to signify thanks for bringing them through a harvest, a life passage, or a terrible occasion. As you dance around your home, remember how far you've come. Dancing conjures up positive, inner peace and power, and changes your mood positively. If you feel a little drama coming your way, then dance and feel good to relieve the stress. Dance around the room. Let the music groove and move you. Feel good. Feel good about yourself. Dance. Dance. Dance.

every minute offers an opportunity for us to learn more about ourselves.

After all, I started as a meat eater, and then became a vegetarian, and am now a vegan with raw food tendencies! I am currently studying for my certification as a raw vegan lifestyle coach and chef. I've increased the length and intensity of my yoga and meditation practices. I went from exercising rarely to walking daily to hiking, backpacking, running races, and then even returning to childhood games such as jumping rope. Each day, I work toward becoming the person I want to be—the someone I *need* to be. I have become an active-ist and an activist—some-

DRAMA-FREE EXERCISE FOR THE BODY

Of course, dancing is a great form of exercise. Incorporate dancing into your exercise routine. Many exercise videos are based on dance moves to melt away the fat, as well as acquire and maintain a toned body. Dancing gets your heart pumping and increases your cardiovascular endurance. There's no need to go to a club. Turn your music up in your home, and make your living room or bedroom your dance floor. You don't need a partner. Dance with yourself and dance to your own tune.

one who lives for today, does not regret yesterday, and works for a better tomorrow.

Even as my father received his diagnosis of pancreatic cancer, one of my aunts died young of conditions complicated by diabetes, and a tornado knocked at my backdoor, I continued to do my "praise dance." I don't believe you came this far to leave this lifestyle at one month: get your "praise dance" on.

DRAMA-FREE EASY RECIPE

you can do it chapati bread

VEGAN

Celebrate what you can and have done! Make your own chapati bread to accompany delicious Indian meals or use as a wrap for your lunch at work. Chapatis are flat unleavened breads that are ubiquitous in India and Africa. They're used mostly to scoop up stews, but can also be used as breads to hold spreads and sandwiches such as the falafel balls from Day 26. I also use chapatis to accompany my homemade stews and soups, and as a wrap for my lunchtime meals.

Chapatis are a great replacement for breads because they use only water, wheat flour, and a little olive oil. I make mine vegan friendly by not using ghee, or clarified butter, which is often employed in Indian cuisine. Chapatis are healthful, quick, inexpensive, and easy to make. It takes ten to fifteen minutes to mix the dough and in another twenty minutes you have ten to twelve chapatis.

Preparation Time: 10–15 minutes to mix the dough
Cooking Time: 20 minutes
Servings: 10–12 chapattis
Storage: I keep extra chapatis in a freezer bag in my refrigerator, and warm them up during the week to accompany stews or as wraps for lunches. Chapatis keep fresh for a week in the refrigerator in a gallon freezer-storage bag.

Ingredients

2 1/4 cup whole-wheat flour

1/2 tsp sea salt

1 cup water

1/2 cup or more wheat flour for dusting

Olive oil as needed (in recipe below for kneading dough, and lightly oiling pan for cooking on the stovetop)

Directions

1. In a large mixing bowl, add the flour and salt.
2. Make a well in the bowl, and add the water.
3. Mix with your hands until you have a smooth and flexible dough.
4. Dust a cutting board with wheat flour, and place the dough on the board.
5. Oil your hands lightly with olive oil, and kneed the dough on the board.
6. Divide the dough into ten to twelve equal pieces and form balls.
7. Flatten each ball individually on the board, and shape each ball with a rolling pin into a six-inch circumference.
8. Heat a frying pan with a small amount of olive oil (2 tsp should do it or more if needed to lightly coat pan), and cook chapatis one at a time in the pan for one minute on each side.
9. Place chapatis on a plate as they are done, and cover with a cloth. Serve warm.

DAY 29

always smile

I've talked about maintaining a positive attitude and chilling out and having fun. I've also mentioned that it's good to smile. Why? Because smiling brings positive energy and gives you hope. Why be angry when this vegetarian journey has done so many positive things for your life? Smiling illustrates to yourself and others how thankful you are for another chance to be healthy. It encourages others to smile with you and calms and relaxes you and them.

Of course, I don't mean that you should walk around with a forced smirk on your face. But it's true that occasionally deliberately willing yourself to smile will actually change your mood—and that of people around you—for the better. I never knew anyone who remained literally down-in-the-mouth when they lifted their facial muscles into a smile.

You made it thus far by faith, strength, endurance, love for your-

DRAMA-FREE MIND AND SPIRIT EXERCISES

If you don't want drama in your home, workplace, or anywhere, then smile. If someone makes you mad, take several deep breaths, think before you react, and keep smiling inwardly and outwardly. When you become angry and want revenge, you use more energy and often end up hurting yourself more than the object of your anger. You experience skyrocketing blood pressure, stress, anxiety, nervousness, and negativity. What a waste of time and energy! Don't create this drama in your life. You can instead turn the negative energy into a positive force to heal yourself and your relationship with others. Maya Angelou put it best when she said, "If you have only one smile in you, give it to the people you love. Don't be surly at home, then go out in the street and start grinning 'Good morning' at total strangers."

self, and determination. You've resisted those who've tried to bring you down, turn you into something you're not—or not yet—and ignored those who are envious of your new lifestyle. You have soared and sailed above adversity, and you've picked yourself up when you stumbled and got back on the path. Now you have the fortitude to carry on. You deserve to give yourself love by smiling right back at yourself.

One way to start your day smiling is by laughing. On many mornings, I skip listening to or watching the news, and watch a comedian on TV, or DVD, or the Internet. Sometimes I switch up different comedians every week or daily, as I relax with my oatmeal and a cup of coffee. You can read a funny book or even make yourself laugh using the techniques called laughter yoga. As the famous *Reader's Digest* column has it, laughter really is the best medicine. When we learn to laugh and laugh at ourselves, we find inner peace and can deal with our drama directly.

DRAMA-FREE EASY RECIPE

make me smile spicy-chunky spanish gazpacho soup

VEGAN

I love soups. Soups are quick, one-pot meals that basically cook by themselves once the ingredients have been added. My love of soups extends throughout all four seasons. However, on those hundred-degree days, when all I want to do is cool down with a quick after-work meal, Spanish gazpacho soup is a perfect way to do so. You can prepare this soup even more quickly than hummus, which only takes ten minutes in a food processor! Although gazpacho is a soup that's traditionally served cold, I've heated this soup up after storing leftovers in the freezer and it's just as good. Whether served hot or cold, gazpacho is delicious and quick, and makes me smile. As long as I have soup, I'm happy all year round!

Ingredients

1 large cucumber, chopped (leave skin on)

3 garlic cloves, minced

1/2 tsp ground chipotle pepper

1 cup green peppers, chopped

1 cup onions, chopped

1 cup mustard greens, chopped roughly

1 cup corn

2 14 1/2-oz. can diced fired-roasted tomatoes

1 46-oz. bottle Spicy Hot V8 juice

1 15 1/2-oz. can black beans, rinsed and drained

1 15 1/2-oz. can red beans, rinsed and drained

1 tsp Bragg's Liquid Aminos

2 tbsp raw apple cider vinegar

Directions

1. Mix all ingredients in a large mixing bowl with a wooden spoon.
2. Serve in individual bowls with Day 9 Spicy Mexican Cornbread.
3. Serving suggestion: Place a dollop of vegan sour cream or plain organic yogurt on top of each soup serving.

DAY 30

congratulations! a summary of drama-free mind, body, and spirit vegetarian living

Congratulations! Take a bow. Give yourself flowers. Wrap your arms around yourself, and give yourself a hug! You've made it through a whole month and the journey is going to get even better. You've avoided the mess, the stress, and the drama. You've taken your small steps and set (and reset) your goals and you've completed thirty days.

It's okay to get emotional; it's okay to praise yourself—because you deserve it. Tell yourself: "It's an honor to be here on this earth, living a healthy and zestful life!" You have added extra years to your life by taking your steps toward better health.

DRAMA-FREE MIND AND SPIRIT EXERCISES

1. Look back on the journal you've been keeping for your vegetarian path.
2. Use what you've written and learned as a means of inspiration, motivation, and empowerment. Reflect on when you were depressed, wanted to go back to eating meat, or felt as though everything didn't seem to be going your way—and see how, in spite of the storms, you've come this far. By looking back at what you've achieved, you can recommit yourself to going forward. You have the energy and the foundation to keep you on the joyous, wondrous path of possibilities and health.

DRAMA-FREE EXERCISE FOR THE BODY

1. Don't let your exercise program stop here. Continue with it, adding new routines. Mix it up with fun games such as running races, dodgeball, or softball on your church team or at family gatherings.
2. Remember to be childlike and enjoy the activity. Exercise is not a chore. It provides a foundation for a better tomorrow—*your* tomorrow.
3. Note in your journal if you've lost weight. Even if your goal isn't to lose weight, use the journal to note how strong and healthy you are through exercise. An exercise journal also provides motivation and inspiration for you to continue. It's a living testament to your progress: how far you've come, and where you're going.

on another journey
sautéed heirloom vegetables

VEGAN

One month as a vegetarian! You've tried new exercises and meals; you've traveled to different countries in your kitchen and discovered who you are. In celebration of this new lifestyle and newfound you, here's a recipe using heirloom produce that you rarely see in local groceries but can be found at your local farmers' market. You can also easily grow your own heirloom produce. These are found locally and inexpensively. Your local farmer is just waiting for your support. This is an opportunity to discover your local farmer and take this journey to another level.

Servings: 2–4
Cooking and Preparation Time: approximately 15 minutes

Ingredients

Wheat or quinoa pasta of choice

2 tbsp olive oil

Heirloom produce: chocolate bell pepper, sliced finger eggplant, sliced rosa bianca eggplant, sliced ghost eggplant

1 large onion

4 garlic cloves, sliced thin

Garlic salt

Black pepper to taste

Directions

1. Cook pasta according to package directions.
2. Meanwhile, heat olive oil in a large pan.
3. Sauté vegetables with onions and garlic for five to eight minutes, or until just tender.
4. Season with garlic salt and black pepper to taste.
5. Plate pasta. Drizzle olive oil on pasta. Place sautéed vegetables on top.
6. Serve with crusty, warmed Italian bread of choice, drizzled in olive oil.

DAY 31

live long and prosper

*"The world is before you and you need not take it
or leave it as it was when you came in."*

—JAMES A. BALDWIN

Day 31 is a bonus day. This will be the start of the second month or, if there are thirty-one days in the month you started this journey, you'll have completed a full month! Are you ready to live the rest of the year and upcoming years drama free? Remember what you've learned, and practice it daily!

To keep you focused, I've included my "Sister Vegetarian's Energy Bar" tips. These energy bars are ten powerful points of focus and meditation to follow daily on your vegetarian or vegan path. If you follow these points, they'll uplift you and give you the fuel you need to continue. I call them "energy bars" because, just like the physical sticks of chewy glucose bars you eat, Sister's Energy Bars offer nutritious and fulfilling ingredients to nourish your mind and body—with an extra dosage of spirit. I encourage you to mentally consume all ten energy bars daily as you walk your path. They'll empower you, and encourage you to continue on your journey.

Why should the spirit be an important ingredient? Because while we're taking care of our bodies, we need to look after our souls. What good is taking back our health if we return to a poor attitude if something or someone gets us down? We juggle many things (family, children, jobs, cooking, cleaning . . . and that's just one day). Are we too tired to remember to take care of ourselves? Are we letting work pull us down and control our lives, rather than us controlling work and how we choose to respond when work becomes overbearing? We need to keep our minds and spirits just as healthy as our bodies. Even if you've been a vegetarian for decades, you need to practice something that renews and empowers your mind and spirit. When we take care of the *entire package* of body, mind, and spirit, we're able to take on whatever challenges us.

sister vegetarian's energy bars

Ingredients
Ten varieties of nutritious and filling ingredients to nourish your mind, body, and spirit, to live successfully as a vegetarian or vegan.

Directions
Consume all ten bars daily for positive fuel as you walk your vegetarian or vegan path.

Energy Bar 1: Be Thankful

When I get up, I thank and praise God for another day. I ask him to surround me with the power and tools I need to meet life's daily challenges and joys. It doesn't matter what religion you practice or whether you practice any religion at all, but it's always good to thank your God, Mother Earth, or the Universe for the day that's been brought forth. Give thanks for the health you're making better (or have made better) through a vegetarian or vegan diet. Give thanks for having shelter, food on your table, clothes on your back, and another day to make right what wasn't made right yesterday—another day to start over, to smile, to rejoice in this life and be exceedingly glad (as Matthew 5:12 puts it) that you've made it this far through trials and tribulations. Thank the Source that you were able to brush yourself off after you fell on your face, stand up straight, and walk away with your shoulders straight and head held high, because crying lasts only but a night and joy comes in the morning (as Psalm 30 has it)! Thank the divine because through faith you know things will happen. Give thanks for the gift of the rain, the sunshine, and the strength that comes from nowhere and gives you the power to do what needs to be done.

Energy Bar 2: Dance for Joy and to Celebrate Life

When I get out of bed at five a.m., I exercise before I prepare myself for work. I listen to songs of empowerment as I ride my stationary bike or do my yoga practice. Afterward, I dance to a song of empowerment. I dance to smile and renew my mind and spirit, since I've taken care of my body through exercise and my vegan diet. Whether you dance to a slow or fast song, give yourself your time. This is your dance of life.

Energy Bar 3: Keep the Faith and Don't Give Up!

Two vital ingredients: faith and endurance. Keep faith in what you can accomplish and don't give up when the going gets tough in any or all aspects of your life. We all have talents and gifts that are different. Just because it may be different, your position, dream, or idea isn't less worthy than that of your sibling. If you can't love yourself through self-motivation, then no one else will motivate you.

Energy Bar 4: You Can't Lose with the Stuff I Use!

Some of you may remember Rev. Frederick Eikerenkoetter, the Pentecostal preacher more commonly known as "Reverend Ike." His favorite slogan was, "You can't lose with the stuff I use!" He'd ask people to send him money and he'd give them a blessing. My grandmother, along with many grandmothers in the early 1970s, it seems, loved Reverend Ike. Well, I'm not asking you to send me money (!), but I do believe that you can't lose with the plant-based diet I propose. I fully believe that this lifestyle will heal your body as you take back your health, and it will provide you with ultimate health benefits as you become a seasoned vegetarian and vegan. The slogan is also a very effective rejoinder to anyone who's giving you a hard time. I can't promise they'll have a spiritual revelation, but I guarantee they'll stop bothering you and you'll be able to walk away from a potential energy-sapping confrontation without wasting your breath.

Energy Bar 5: Stand!

Susie is trying to lose weight. A coworker likes to talk about losing weight, but she doesn't have a plan, and so wallows in self-pity. She sees Susie and is envious. She decides to sabotage Susie's plan by constantly asking her to join her for a piece of chocolate cake, a donut, cookie, or lunch at a fast-food restaurant. Those who are unhappy with their lifestyle will do anything to bring others down because, well, misery loves company. These drama queens and kings want you to fall—and they'll get you when you yourself may be at your most vulnerable or lowest. This is the time to dust yourself off, hold your head up high, stick out your chest, jump over that hole you or someone else decided to dig for you, and stand up tall. Do it while you're reading this. It feels energizing and empowering, doesn't it? It feels good to be in control when you take a stand. So, *stand!*

Energy Bar 6: Victory!

As I wrote at the beginning of this book, you were victorious from Day 1. Claim that victory through recognizing how you're healing your body and reducing your dependence on pharmaceuticals and medical procedures.

Energy Bar 7: Rise!

There's a famous painting by Annie Lee called *Blue Monday*. It shows a woman sitting hunched on the bed, as if the last thing she wants to do is get up and get going. I'd love to tell the woman depicted that if she knew that she could rise through the trials and tribulations, as well as the good times, and that the sun shines even on cloudy days, she wouldn't be so depressed. I'd tell her that Mondays come and go, and cannot control what's in her heart, mind, and spirit. Of course, we all have the Monday blues, but I won't let them determine my life. I *rise* and stand above Mondays. I *rise* and stand above drama, depression, sadness, and all thoughts toxic to my being. I call upon my vegetarian and vegan sisters and brothers to do the same. Be the master of your vessel and *rise* to meet the challenge.

Energy Bar 8: Testify!

We are walking testaments to taking back our health. Write your own. Testify to all of the joy you're experiencing, so others can also learn to take back their health. Keep a journal or post it where you can see it daily. Remind yourself of where you've been and where you are going.

Energy Bar 9: Open the Door

You have everything you need to succeed as a vegetarian and vegan. You have the knowledge and tools. All you need to do is take the step to maintain a healthy body, mind, and spirit. Being a vegetarian and vegan is not only about abstaining from eating animal products. It's a lifestyle of vegetables, proteins, and complex carbs, exercise, and a positive attitude. You hold the key to good health, so just open the door and take a step in the right direction.

Energy Bar 10: Do Not Be Hard on Yourself

We may be on the right path, but we're always works in progress. This is a lifelong journey where tomorrow is always a day ahead—for ten, twenty, even fifty years from now. You are bringing vitality and strength to your golden years by working today with a vegetarian or vegan lifestyle. Mentally and spiritually, you're also growing in different ways. Who knows? You may become an activist in your community, working today to change tomorrow's path for yourself and others.

I hope these Energy Bars continue to inspire,
empower, and uplift you through your journey.

—SISTER VEGETARIAN

red quinoa, lentils, and farro cakes

By Chef Ricky Moore

Vegetarian and Vegan

For the final recipe in this book, I want to inspire you to find ingredients you've never tried as a vegetarian. I want you to become motivated to seek out the endless possibilities of creating meals at home that stimulate all your senses with ingredients that are both easily accessible and new to you. This recipe will not only inspire and motivate you, but leave you licking your fingers, lips, and plate for more! Trust me, this is exactly what happened when Chef Ricky Moore prepared this dish in a vegetarian cooking class. I had no shame! It was good!

Two of Chef Ricky's favorite quotes illustrate his love of incorporating fresh, natural foods into our lifestyles:

Nothing will benefit human health and increase the chances for survival of life on Earth as much as the evolution to a vegetarian diet.

—ALBERT EINSTEIN (ATTRIBUTED)

I liked the fresh, pure tastes of natural foods; but even more important, I liked the glowing feeling of health, vigor and energy which followed my change in diet.

—DICK GREGORY

Preparation Time: 1 hour
Servings: 22 3-oz. cakes

Ingredients

4 1/2 cups vegetable stock, divided

8 ounces red quinoa

8 ounces farro

7 ounces firm tofu

7 ounces cooked red lentils, puréed

1 red onion, minced

Olive oil, as needed for searing

5 cloves garlic, minced

1/2 cup fresh chopped cilantro

1/2 cup fresh chopped parsley

2 tablespoons chipotle powder

1 tablespoon cumin, ground

1 tablespoon coriander, ground

Panko bread crumbs, as needed

Salt and black pepper, to taste

Directions

1. In a pot, bring 2 cups vegetable stock to a boil. Meanwhile, rinse the red quinoa. Add to boiling stock and cook, uncovered, for fifteen minutes.

2. In a separate pot, bring 2 cups stock to a boil and cook farro, uncovered, for twenty-five to thirty minutes.

3. Purée 1 cup cooked farro, just enough to leave a little consistency.

4. Purée the tofu and lentils; add to the puréed farro. In a pan, sauté onions in olive oil until translucent, and fold into the mixture.

5. In a bowl, combine the puréed farro/tofu-lentil, the rest of the cooked farro, cooked quinoa, the remaining vegetable stock, garlic, cilantro, parsley, chipotle powder, cumin, and coriander. Mix well. (If mixture is too wet, add just enough Panko bread crumbs to enhance binding.)

6. Season with salt and pepper.
7. Portion out burger mix into 3-oz. patties.
8. Lightly coat each patty with Panko.
9. Pan-sear each patty in olive oil for three minutes per side.

> *Note:* I would recommend making your favorite homemade condiment, such as Thousand Island dressing (vegetarian recipe), cilantro pesto, and red cabbage relish.

Chef Ricky Moore was the 2007 Iron Chef America Warrior in Food Network's 2007 Iron Chef America Thanksgiving Special. Chef Ricky Moore has a wealth of national and international cooking experience, including as executive chef at top restaurants and hotels in the Washington, D.C., Chicago, and New York City areas. Chef Ricky has also traveled to France, Toronto, and Singapore to work as a chef. Chef Ricky's culinary influence stems from a mixture of his North Carolina upbringing, modern French cuisine, and the many cooks of his family and other chefs, who believe in incorporating foods in season and love preparing food. You can visit Chef Ricky at his website www.chefrickymoore.com.

rights of passage reborn

TASHI S. WINSTON

Coming out of darkness to now see the light
As a haze that glows over the pain that once was there
A new day arises for you and baptizes you in a river of purifying glory
You are on your way to a better start than you ever thought before
No more tears, lost breath of undistinguished
fears knocking at your nerves
Tears that you once cried out, full of confusion and disparity
Now dried up and uplifted to a better day
Illumines words uttered from my mouth unmentioned
Hands and feet reborn blissfully in Gods eyes
Beauty and clarity surfaces you as a glimpse of hope and love
Covering you like a blanket that bestows you with a breath of fresh air
No words can ever be spoken to an emancipated heart with knowledge
Under wings floating and flying with peace
A new day has come
Songs of happiness spill out of your veins like a mystical flower
A new moon has grown

The blessing of a new body is evolving

Turning into a brand-new being

Leaving behind what was and walking toward what is

The world is your baby your lover and your heart. . . .

With each breath you take in tasteful sighs

Grabbing each and every fruitful bite that it has to offer

Smiling at the happiness that it has to offer you

Never thought I would get here,

So happy and free in a cool spirit abundantly bright

Bright as the light that once shone me serenity

Laying down laws to fit my own lifestyle

I'm flawless in my own right. . .

Yes this woman right here. . .

Having grace, style, and divine words

Coming into my exclusive power trip that is handled maturely

No more waiting for someone to serve me

Digesting unequal rights that fell at my side like confetti

It is my destiny to be free . . . to be free to be free.

And let my life truly be.

what's in sister vegetarian's pantry?

O r should the question be, What can Sister not do without when preparing my weekly vegan meals? I always keep on hand certain staples, so I'm always able to create a dish. Of course, once a week I'll purchase one or more items from my farmers' market, or whole foods or grocery store to make a meal I've never made or rarely make. But because I love to cook and create beautiful and loving vegan meals in my kitchen, I need to have some essentials on hand. (Many of the items I've listed below can be purchased in bulk and fresh.)

Various Vegan Milks

Rice milk

Hemp milk

Almond milk

Canned coconut milk (makes a great Indian curry sauce)

Beans and Legumes

Garbanzo beans (aka chickpeas), canned and dry

Turtle beans (aka black beans), canned and dry

Lentil beans (green, yellow, and if they can be found, red), dry

Kidney beans (canned and dry)

Great northern beans (canned)

Cannellini beans (canned)

16-bean dry bean (package)

Green or yellow split peas (dry)

Cranberry beans (dry)

Black-eyed peas (dry)

Adzuki beans (dry)

Fresh Greens

Collards

Beet greens

Kale

Turnip greens

Red chard/Swiss chard

Beet roots

Other Fresh Produce and Soy Products

Tofu

Onions (white and/or yellow)

Garlic (I am a garlic fanatic. Give me six to eight cloves in any meals and I'm happy.)

Organic carrots

Sweet potatoes and white potatoes (although I don't use them often, I immediately cut up after purchase and freeze to always have on hand for stews or vegan fries).

Eggplant (I slice in half-inch to one-inch rounds as soon as I purchase and freeze. These make great grilled sandwiches for a quick after-work meal.)

Tomatoes (great in sandwiches and tortilla wraps)

Apples (an apple a day with my work-time lunches)

Bananas (a banana a day as a midmorning snack)

Nuts, Grains, Raisins, Wheat, Cornmeal

Quinoa

Farro

Bulgur

Brown rice

Quinoa pasta

Steel-cut oats (I'm in heaven at breakfast time)

Sunflower seeds (to make home-made vegan cheese)

Peanuts (I add this to my steel-cut oats for breakfast; great in African stews and Asian noodle dishes)

Cashews (a great midmorning snack and used to make vegan cheese)

Raisins (I add to my steel-cut oats for breakfast; use as a snack with peanuts for an afternoon work pick-me-up. Also known as GORP—Good Old-Fashioned Raisins and Peanuts—in hiking/backpacking terminology.)

Organic flaxseed (I add to my steel-cut oats for breakfast; also use in homemade vegan breads.)

Wheat tortillas (wraps that can be used in place of chapatis when serving Middle Eastern, Indian, and African stews)

Organic cornmeal (great in making vegan cornbread to accompany Mexican and South American bean stews and soups)

Spices, Peppers, Condiments, Miscellaneous

Organic Raw Apple Cider Vinegar

Bragg's Organic 24 Seasonings

Bragg's Liquid Aminos

Vegan liquid smoke

Nutritional yeast

Parsley (dried)

Basil (dried and fresh)

Oregano (dried)

Thyme (dried)

Sea Salt

Black pepper

Red pepper flakes

Cumin (ground)

Turmeric (ground)

Curry powder

Cinnamon, allspice, nutmeg, ginger (ground—I grouped these together because they're essentials in Indian, Caribbean, and some African meals. A combination of the three is also a foundation of a jerk seasoning)

Paprika (smoked and regular)

Tamarind paste

Chipotle peppers (ground)

Chipotle peppers in Adobo sauce

Chili pepper (ground)

Jalapeño peppers (fresh)

Habanero peppers (fresh)

Cubanelle peppers (fresh)

Lavender (fresh)

Rosemary (fresh)

Tahini (used in my weekly hummus spread for lunch; and to make tahini dressing, which I love on my raw/live greens salads)

Organic peanut butter

Vegan mayonnaise

Vegan sour cream

Extra virgin olive oil (A major asset for my kitchen. I need to invest in stock for olive oil and garlic!)

Yeast packets (to make homemade vegan bread)

Lemon juice

Lemons (fresh)

Soy sauce

Organic maple syrup (great for making the dressing for the live collards salad)

Corn starch (great for thickening Asian sauces)

Baking soda

Organic raw sugar

Gallon white vinegar (for making your own vegetable wash—2 tbsp per 2 cups water in a spray bottle or in a tub)

Assorted teas and coffees

Bon Appétit
—Sister Vegetarian

additional resources: documentaries and books

These lists will educate you in order to make better choices, take back your health, and continue on a lifelong vegetarian journey.

Documentaries

Forks over Knives
(www.forksoverknives.com)

Food Matters
(www.foodmatters.tv)

The Gerson Miracle
(www.gerson.org)

The Beautiful Truth
(www.gerson.org)

King Corn
(www.kingcorn.net)

Food, Inc.
(www.foodincmovie.com)

The Future of Food
(www.thefutureoffood.com)

What's on Your Plate?
(www.whatsonyourplatepro
ject.org)

Change Your Food, Change Your Life (www.vegan-gal.com)

Books

Animal Liberation: A New Ethics for our Treatment of Animals by Peter Singer: Ecco, 2002.

By Any Greens Necessary: A Revolutionary Guide for Black Women Who Want to Eat Great, Get Healthy, Lose Weight, and Look Phat by Tracye Lynn McQuirter: Lawrence Hill Books, 2010

The China Study: The Most Comprehensive Study of Nutrition Ever Conducted and the Startling Implications for Diet, Weight Loss and Long-term Health by T. Colin Campbell, Thomas M. Campbell II, Howard Lyman, and John Robbins: Ben Bella Books, 2005.

Disposable People: New Slavery in the Global Economy by Kevin Bales: University of California Press, 2000.

The Dreaded Comparison: Human and Animal Slavery by Marjorie Spiegel (foreword by Alice Walker): Mirror Books, 1997.

Healing the Gerson Way: Defeating Cancer and Other Chronic Diseases by Charlotte Gerson, Beata Bishop, Joanne Shwed, and Robert Stone: Totality Books, 2007.

Food Inc.: A Participant Guide: How Industrial Food Is Making Us Sicker, Fatter, and Poorer— And What You Can Do About It by Participant Media and Karl Weber: Public Affairs, 2009.

How to Eat like a Vegetarian Even if You Never Want to Be One by Carol J. Adams and Patti Breitman: Lantern Books, 2008.

Living with Meat Eaters: The Vegetarian's Survival Handbook by Carol J. Adams: Lantern Books, 2008.

Genetic Roulette: The Documented Health Risks of Genetically Engineered Foods by Jeffrey M. Smith: Chelsea Green, 2007.

Natural Diet for Folks Who Eat: Cookin' with Mother Nature by Dick Gregory: HarperCollins, 1983.

Seeds of Deception: Exposing Industry and Government Lies about the Safety of the Genetically Engineered Foods You're Eating by Jeffrey M. Smith: Yes! Books, 2003.

Sistah Vegan: Black Female Vegans Speak on Food, Identity,

Health, and Society, edited by A. Breeze Harper: Lantern Books, 2010.

Skinny Bitch by Rory Freedman and Kim Barnouin: Running Press, 2005.

Veganomicon: The Ultimate Vegan Cookbook by Isa Chandra Moskowitz and Terry Hope Romero: Marlowe & Co., 2007.

Vegan Soul Kitchen: Fresh, Healthy, and Creative African-American Cuisine by Bryant Terry: Da Capo, 2009.

The Vegan Cook's Bible by Pat Crocker: Robert Rose, 2009.

The Vegetarian Bible: The Complete Illustrated Guide to Vegetarian Food & Cooking by Sarah Brown: Reader's Digest, 2002.

sister vegetarian's drama-free goals chart

Walk your vegetarian or vegan journey step by step and day by day. Small steps lead to a bigger journey! Goals can help you maintain a vegetarian or vegan lifestyle by building your confidence. Through setting and reaching goals, "Yes, I Can!" becomes a daily reality.

If you want to live a happy life,
tie it to a goal, not to people or things.
—ALBERT EINSTEIN

	Goal	Start Date	Goal Reached Date	Give yourself a "star" My shining star!
1	Victory! I am a vegetarian—Day 1			
2	1 week as a vegetarian—Loving it!			
3	2 weeks as a vegetarian—I am strong!			
4	3 weeks as a vegetarian—I feel alive!			
5	4 weeks as a vegetarian—I know I can!			
6	31 days as a vegetarian—You go, girl!			
7				
8				
9				
10				
11				
12				
13				
14				
15				
16				
17				
18				
19				
20				

sister's weekly menu planner

One of the keys to a drama-free vegetarian and vegan lifestyle is meal planning. When you know what's on the menu and what's accessible to you on a daily basis, preparing and eating healthy meals becomes less time consuming. It doesn't feel like a chore but like fun, instead; and the age-old question of "What should I eat?" becomes a statement of the past.

	Sunday	Monday	Tuesday	Wednesday	Thursday	Friday	Saturday
Breakfast							
Snack							
Lunch							
Snack							
Dinner							
Dessert; Tea							